Research Skills for Medical Students

Research Skills for **Medical Students**

Editor:
Ann K. Allen

Series Editors:
Judy McKimm and Kirsty Forrest

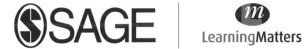

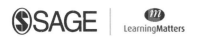

Learning Matters
An imprint of Sage Publications Ltd
1 Oliver's Yard
55 City Road
London EC1Y 1SP

SAGE Publications Inc
2455 Teller Road
Thousand Oaks, California 91320

Sage Publications India Pvt Ltd
B 1/I 1 Mohan Cooperative Industrial Area
Mathura Road
New Delhi 110 044

SAGE Publications Asia-Pacific Pte Ltd
3 Church Street
#10-04 Samsung Hub
Singapore 049483

Editor: Becky Taylor
Development editor: Ros Morley
Production controller: Chris Marke
Project management: Swales & Willis Ltd,
Exeter, Devon
Marketing manager: Tamara Navaratnam
Cover and text design: Code 5 Design Associates
Typeset by: Swales & Willis Ltd, Exeter, Devon
Printed by: MPG Books Group, Bodmin, Cornwall

First published 2012

Library of Congress Control Number:
2012938955

British Library Cataloguing in Publication data

A catalogue record for this book is available
from the British Library

ISBN 978-0-85725-837-3
ISBN 978-0-85725-601-0 (pbk)

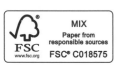

Contents

Foreword from the Series Editors

The Learning Matters Medical Education Series

Medical education is currently experiencing yet another a period of change, typified in the UK with the introduction of the revised *Tomorrow's Doctors* (General Medical Council, 2009) and ongoing work on establishing core curricula for many subject areas. Changes are also occurring at Foundation and postgraduate levels in terms of the introduction of broader non-technical competencies, a wider range of assessments and revalidation requirements. This new series of textbooks has been developed as a direct response to these changes and the impact on all levels of medical education.

Research indicates that effective medical practitioners combine excellent, up-to-date clinical and scientific knowledge with practical skills and the ability to work with patients, families and other professionals with empathy and understanding; they know when to lead and when to follow and they work collaboratively and professionally to improve health outcomes for individuals and communities. In *Tomorrow's Doctors*, the General Medical Council has defined a series of learning outcomes set out under three headings:

1. The doctor as a scholar and a scientist;
2. The doctor as a practitioner;
3. The doctor as a professional.

The books in this series do not cover practical clinical procedures or knowledge about diseases and conditions, but instead cover the range of non-technical professional skills (plus underpinning knowledge) that students and doctors need to know in order to become effective, safe and competent practitioners.

Aimed specifically at medical students (but also of use for Foundation doctors, teachers and clinicians), each book relates to specific outcomes of *Tomorrow's Doctors* (and, where relevant, the Foundation curriculum), providing both knowledge and help to improve the skills necessary to be successful at the non-clinical aspects of training as a doctor. One of the aims of the series is to set medical practice within the wider social, policy and organisational agendas to help produce future doctors who are socially aware and willing and prepared to engage in broader issues relating to healthcare delivery.

Individual books in the series outline the key theoretical approaches and policy agendas relevant to that subject, and go further by demonstrating through case studies and scenarios how these theories can be used in work settings to achieve best practice. Plenty of activities and self-assessment tools throughout the book will help readers to hone their critical thinking and reflection skills.

Chapters in each of the books follow a standard format. At the beginning a box highlights links to relevant competencies and outcomes from *Tomorrow's Doctors* and other medical curricula, if appropriate. This sets the scene and enables readers to see exactly what will be covered. This is extended by a chapter overview which sets out the key topics and what students should expect to have learnt by the end of the chapter.

There is at least one case study in each chapter which considers how theory can be used in practice from different perspectives. Activities are included which include practical tasks with learning points, critical thinking research tasks and reflective practice/thinking points. Activities can be carried out by readers or with others and are designed to raise awareness, consolidate understanding of theories and ideas and enable students to improve their practice by using models, approaches and ideas. Each activity is followed by a brief discussion on issues raised. At the end of each chapter a chapter summary provides an aide-mémoire of what has been covered.

All chapters are evidence-based in that they set out the theories or evidence that underpins practice. In most chapters, one or more 'What's the evidence?' boxes provide further information about a particular piece of research or a policy agenda through books, articles, websites or policy papers. A list of additional readings is set out under the 'Going further' section, with all references collated at the end of the book.

The series is edited by Professor Judy McKimm and Dr Kirsty Forrest, both of whom are experienced medical educators and writers. Book and chapter authors are drawn from a wide pool of practising clinicians and educators from the UK and internationally.

About the Authors

Ann Allen is a Senior Lecturer in the Institute of Medical Education, Cardiff University. Previously Director of Cardiff University's Master of Public Health Programme, Ann trained initially in sociology and anthropology and has worked in many developing countries as well as acting as an adviser to health-related projects for the UK Department of International Development, and for international agencies in Africa, South America and Commonwealth of Independent States (CIS). As well as teaching global health to medical students she contributes to an open education initiative peoples-uni (www.peoples-uni.org) that supports the continuous professional development of doctors and others working in public health.

Seema Biswas is a general surgeon, Red Cross Health Delegate and lecturer in surgery and global health. She has taught medical students for over 15 years and works with students on research projects, especially in medical education and global health. As Lead Clinical Editor for *onExamination* – from BMJ Learning she collaborated with Ann Allen in 2011 in teaching an SSC in Global health and medical education.

Dawn Lau has worked as a Clinical Teaching Fellow at the Cardiff School of Medicine and has been a registrar in Respiratory Medicine at the Cardiff and Vale University Health Board. She is involved both in undergraduate and postgraduate medical education and her range of educational endeavours include organisation of a pilot peer-assisted learning programme in clinical skills within the undergraduate core curriculum, developing assessment schemes for the student selected components (SSCs) and running the formal educational programme for the Core Medical Trainees (CMTs) within the Health Board. She has recently become Consultant in Respiratory Medicine/Cystic Medicine in Cardiff.

Blanche Lumb and *Michael Hollifield* carried out initial coding of 24 transcripts of student feedback encounters. These were encounters where pairs of medical students presented patients they had seen to consultants in a variety of medical specialties. This work (made possible by a grant from the Cardiff University Research Opportunities Programme) is being carried in collaboration between Professor Charlotte Rees, University of Dundee, College of Medicine, Dentistry & Nursing, Dundee and Dr Lynn Monrouxe and Dr Andrew Grant, Institute of Medical Education, School of Medicine, Cardiff University.

Acknowledgements

The support given from the inception of this book by Dr Sharon Mayor, Senior Lecturer in Healthcare Improvement, Institute of Primary Care & Public Health Cardiff University, is gratefully acknowledged.

The author and publisher would like to thank the following for permission to reproduce copyright material:

BMJ Books/Wiley-Blackwell for excerpt from *How to Read a Paper: The basics of evidence-based medicine*, 4th edition.

Learning Matters (Sage) for Table 2.1 and Figure 4.1 from McKimm, J and Forrest, K (2011) *Professional Practice for Foundation Doctors*. Exeter.

Journal of the American Society for Information Science and Technology for Table 5.3 from Meho, LI (2006) E-mail interviewing in qualitative research: a methodological discussion. *Journal of the American Society for Information Science and Technology*, 57(10): 1284–95.

Every effort has been made to trace all copyright holders within the book, but if any have been inadvertently overlooked the publisher will be pleased to make the necessary arrangements at the first opportunity.

Introduction
Ann K. Allen

Reading through someone else's research or undertaking a piece of research yourself is an unavoidable and essential part of learning and later practising medicine. We are sure you've heard doctors say that they never stop learning: they read; they study; they watch others work; most importantly, though, when they come across something new they have to decide whether they ought to change the way they work. This is evidence-based medicine, and to understand exactly how big a problem a particular disease is, how risk in lifestyles (e.g. smoking or driving too fast) actually affects disease, how decisions are made to treat diseases in a specific way and whether medical interventions really work, understanding research is key.

This book is written specifically for medical students and Foundation doctors to show you how to:

- make sense of the research and medical literature you read;
- judge the quality of what you are reading and decide whether it's worth acting upon;
- undertake a piece of research on a subject that interests you;
- write research articles and case reports;
- get your research published.

Our aim is that this book will help you develop the critical thinking and research skills that will enable you to become the 'scholars and scientists' in medicine required by *Tomorrow's Doctors* (General Medical Council, 2009) and for doctors in *Good Medical Practice* (General Medical Council, 2006). We try to make sense of the world of medical literature for you (including journals and the wealth of material on the internet from blogs to medical society websites), help you understand levels of evidence (how reliable research findings are in relation to changing your practice as a doctor) so that by the time you've read this book you'll have a good idea how to:

- identify a research question;
- carry out an effective literature search;
- understand the value of medical databases and open internet searches, e.g. Google;
- find work that others have done in the same field that interests you, read their literature, find their websites and contact them;

- check for yourself that you are working on the right lines in your own research plans;

- identify what ethical considerations inform all forms of investigation;

- find help close at hand when starting your own research;

- respond to criticism when someone is looking at your plans, research proposals or your reports;

- undertake your own project and tell others about it.

We help you to understand the basic mechanics of knowledge production and consumption in medicine in general. You'll then be able to make sense of the latest literature providing the evidence used to support a change in a common clinical protocol for instance. The book moves from a discussion about the principles underpinning different research designs, through the basics of data collection and analysis to how to disseminate your research and use your own skills to inform and improve both your own and clinical practice in general.

We accept that the need to publish and present is more pressing now than it has ever been in medical school. We endeavour to give you reasons for this and help you develop a healthy interest in publishing your work. We have also put together a useful list of contacts in medical publishing who are also able to help you on your way. We hope that by the time you come to apply for Foundation or specialty training, you have a couple of publications of your own to display on your application form.

Hopefully both as students and doctors you will not just be consumers of knowledge, but will share your experience and ideas and go on to become teachers and researchers communicating through peer review and, in time, clinicians participating in clinical trials. Some of you will become active scientists in the widening fields that extend beyond the basic physical and social sciences into implementation and evaluation. As trainees and doctors, you will undertake clinical audits and participate in quality improvement initiatives to enhance the service that you offer to your patients.

Underpinning this book is the recognition that 'knowledge' is something that is contingent and changing. Thus understanding research is essential in order to identify how, and to what extent, 'evidence' is to be trusted. Critical thinking is fundamental to medicine: whether in formulating differential diagnoses and interpreting the results of investigations or in understanding how the findings of a study are limited by the way the study is framed (its design, the data collection tools, the population studied and the way in which the results are analysed). Moreover, it's important to recognise how the wider social, cultural and political context in which the research was undertaken and reported influences not only the questions posed but also the interpretation of the results. This book aims therefore not only to explain research skills to you, but also to develop your wider critical thinking skills and awareness of the context of your research.

Background to the book

Three key policy documents provide the rationale for this present book.

1. *Good Medical Practice* (General Medical Council, 2006) identifies the principles and values that are the foundation for good practice for doctors. Medical professionalism is based on these principles. The document *Good Medical Practice* stresses that individuals are personally accountable for their professional practice and that they must always be prepared to justify their decisions and actions. The most defensible justification is on the basis of sound evidence derived from rigorous and systematic investigation. Regarding research specifically it states:

   - *70. Research involving people directly or indirectly is vital in improving care and reducing uncertainty for patients now and in the future, and improving the health of the population as a whole.*

   - *71. If you are involved in designing, organising or carrying out research, you must:*

     ◦ *put the protection of the participants' interests first*

     ◦ *act with honesty and integrity*

     ◦ *follow the appropriate national research governance guidelines and the guidance in* Research: The role and responsibilities of doctors.

Another important principle in this document is to provide a good standard of practice and care. Doing so requires doctors to keep their professional knowledge and skills up to date and participate in audit and quality improvement reviews.

2. The Department of Health (2005) *Research Governance Framework for Health and Social Care* section 1.6 states:

   All service and academic staff, no matter how senior or junior, have a role to play in the conduct of research.

This document spells out the principles that apply generally to research in health and social care. It applies to the full range of research types, contexts and methods. Two key principles are that:

Whatever the context, the interests of research participants come first. Those responsible must be satisfied they have taken all reasonable steps to protect the dignity, rights, safety and wellbeing of participants. We have to be frank about risks, and businesslike about managing them [ii].

Research can be defined as the attempt to derive generalisable new knowledge by addressing clearly defined questions with systematic and rigorous methods. Quality in research depends on those responsible being appropriately qualified, with the skills and experience to use their professional judgement effectively in the delivery of dependable research (paragraph 1.10).

3. Finally *Tomorrow's Doctors* (General Medical Council, 2009) stipulates the outcomes and standards for undergraduate medical education – these are the standards you must meet in order to pass your basic medical degree and become a doctor. The competencies relating to research within the 'Doctor as a Scholar and as a Scientist' section inform the content of this book. Relevant competencies are included at the start of each chapter to help you map the chapter content to what is expected of you.

Book structure and features

Ten chapters follow the sequence in which research methods are commonly taught. Each chapter starts with a chapter overview and ends with a summary of what has been covered together with suggestions for further reading. References and a glossary of the key concepts are given at the end of the book. Key concepts appear in bold text when introduced for the first time and/or when appropriate. In each chapter there are practical activities designed to consolidate your understanding of ideas and techniques which you can do alone or with others. Some activities require access to the internet. Case studies are also included in each chapter to help you see how the principles of research apply in practice.

Chapter 1: Doing research

This chapter discusses the importance of research, how it informs practice, the sorts of research there are and what paradigms underpin their methods and approaches. It gives an overview of the different forms of study design (whether experimental, population or individual focused, or participatory; to generate or test hypotheses, or to evaluate a service or activity for instance). The chapter explains how an investigation's purpose determines the stringency of requirements for gathering and recording data.

You'll see how to find a relevant topic to research and how the research question affects the selection of the study design. The steps in research are signposted, as are different types of research study which are the focus of later chapters in the book.

Chapter 2: Doing a literature review

This chapter helps you to find (and limit) your reading to material that is most useful to you. It explains when and why a literature review is undertaken in the context of evidence-based medicine (EBM) and the Cochrane Collaboration. It outlines the benefits to patients and practitioners that result from undertaking literature reviews. The distinction between reviewing the literature systematically (that is expected of any student in higher education) and undertaking a systematic literature review is explained. It shows how keywords and bibliographic databases are used in reviewing the literature and takes you through the processes of how to conduct a literature review systematically; and how to appraise, analyse, and report the information so retrieved. Often student dissertations are more annotated bibliographies than literature reviews, so the difference between the two is demonstrated.

Chapter 3: Critical appraisal

This chapter examines how to critically appraise the literature you identified in your literature search and explains what is meant by critical appraisal. You are shown how to critically appraise literature of research with different study designs and to use your knowledge of the practical issues associated with data collection to be able to critically appraise the credibility of research. This should help you to be able to apply these skills to your own research when you come to interpret your results and write up your own study.

Chapter 4: Evaluation and research methods

Doing any investigation means you have to understand some of the basic processes that underpin it. The theoretical approach adopted by researchers frequently reflects values and disciplinary background in addition to the research question. To select an appropriate study design you need to understand its strengths and limitations in order to interpret and to critically appraise the significance of the results and this chapter will help you to do this. Both quantitative and qualitative designs commonly used for research in medicine are outlined. The stages and processes of planning a research study are discussed in this chapter. The chapter assesses how political and ethical factors are constantly negotiated in participatory forms of investigation. The role of ethics in research is discussed.

Chapter 5: Data collection and information gathering

This chapter shows you how to identify and exploit a wide range of information sources. Strategies for locating and accessing information are given along with how to judge data quality. This chapter also examines the practicalities of the information gathering tools (laboratory notebooks, interview schedules and questionnaires, field notes, observation guides etc.) used for research.

Chapter 6: Data processing and analysis

Maintaining confidential records in a format where they can be retrieved for analysis requires systematic planning and good records. Whatever the purpose, data analysis involves a mixture of common sense, technical expertise and sheer curiosity. This chapter covers data preparation, constructing a coding frame, measurement and classification, summarising data, data analysis and presenting statistical data clearly.

Chapter 7: Interpreting the implications of research

Once an investigation is completed it is to be hoped that the research question is answered – or it is clear why that outcome is not achieved. The broader implications of a study need to be examined if they are to be translated into actions that will improve the service offered to patients. The rise of translational research (how to make findings from basic research applicable to medical practice), and the changing modes of scientific (and doctor–patient) interaction that technology (the internet, mobile phones for instance) permits, open up spaces for generating and using new knowledge. This chapter explores the implications of these issues for medical students.

The context in which information was created and the context in which you may want to use it may differ and this chapter will explore how to assess the relevance of and uses of information. Material concerns drive what research topics get funding so you need to remain aware of the wider policy context. Research is increasingly governed by concern with 'time-to-market', and to a large extent professional research now is driven by market demand which makes collaboration, team-working and the use of information technology imperative.

Chapter 8: Communicating the outcomes of research and evaluation

Presenting your research is an art in itself – you have to go back to basics about something you have become immersed in, your audience may well vary in age/experience so what you present has to be understandable by all. This chapter explains how to effectively communicate research and critical evaluation outputs to diverse audiences. The protocol regarding academic publications is explained, together with the importance of recognising intellectual property. You'll be shown what to look out for in making presentations, and designing and presenting posters as these are the most traditional initial ways of communicating research. This chapter also explains how to how to write an academic report and how to write a case report for publication.

Chapter 9: Audit

This chapter examines clinical audit and how it is implemented in practice. Medical students often participate in clinical audits and Foundation doctors certainly do, so it is important that you understand the 'bigger picture' it serves. Clinical audit involves the review of healthcare-related activity data against predefined standards or guidelines. Its primary purpose is to improve quality by promoting adherence to standards. Combined with feedback to and education of clinicians and medical students, clinical audit is a tool that enables clinicians (and the teams in which they work) to improve the care they provide to patients, and thus to build clinical effectiveness.

This chapter also introduces key organisations and their place in the audit network and process, including:

- the National Institute for Health and Clinical Excellence (NICE);

- the National Advisory Group on Clinical Audit and Enquiries (NAGCAE);

- the Healthcare Quality Improvement Partnership (HQIP);

- professional societies.

Chapter 10: Doing health service evaluation and quality improvement

This chapter aims to build your understanding of the process of service evaluation and quality improvement (QI) with a step-by-step guide to the basic principles. It shows you where to seek expertise (about policies and standards/guidelines) and the value of sound evaluation for health service improvement. It explains how and why patient safety and evidence-based care are at the heart of QI. Finally, the chapter helps you to develop techniques for promoting change in both the institutional setting and workplace practice.

> *For the students who are the professionals of the future, developing the ability to investigate problems, make judgments on the basis of sound evidence, take decisions on a rational basis, and understand what they are doing and why is vital. Research and inquiry is not just for those who choose to pursue an academic career. It is central to professional life in the twenty-first century.*
>
> (Brew, 2007, p7)

So many medical students have told us 'they expect us to be able to do research but we're not taught it'. Over the years we've seen students, administrators and even clinical teachers struggle with whether a 'project' or 'student selected component' (SSC) is an audit, a health service evaluation or research. The anxiety this uncertainty provokes is palpable – if an investigation is 'research' you are professionally required to seek approval from a relevant ethics committee. This not only extends the time needed for pre-planning the SSC but there is also the possibility that approval may not be granted in time for the work to be undertaken. Because audit, health service evaluation, quality improvement studies and research all take place in similar settings, with similar personnel, collect similar data and use similar analytic tools the difference between them is not transparent to the novice. This book will help you to tell the differences between these types of study and feel confident in how to approach them. Good luck in your studies!

chapter 1
Doing Research
Ann K. Allen

Achieving your medical degree

This chapter will help you to begin to meet the following requirements of *Tomorrow's Doctors* (General Medical Council, 2009).

Outcomes 1 – The doctor as a scholar and a scientist

12. Apply scientific method and approaches to medical research.

   (b) Formulate simple relevant research questions in biomedical science, psychosocial science or population science, and design appropriate studies or experiments to address the questions.

Outcomes 2 – The doctor as a practitioner

19. Use information effectively in a medical context.

   (b) Make effective use of computers and other information systems, including storing and retrieving information.

The chapter will also enable you to meet the UK Foundation Curriculum (Academy of Medical Royal Colleges, 2012) requirements for engaging in and understanding research, audit and evaluation.

Chapter overview

After reading this chapter you will be able to:

- explain what research is and why research is important;
- explain the purposes of doing research;
- develop some strategies to find a topic to research;
- describe the different approaches to research design;
- explain why it is important to think critically;
- explain how the purpose of doing original research differs from investigations such as doing a literature review, a health service evaluation, audit or quality improvement.

Introduction

Well-designed research produces the credible evidence underpinning **evidence-based medicine**. This will be explained in later chapters. Rather than dwelling on principles of statistics we want to show you that study design and method are key in your research. For now, what is important is that you should appreciate that 'finding out' is done for many reasons. Before you start a research project of any kind you should try to be clear about the answers to:

- 'Why am I doing it?'
- 'Why am I doing it this way?'
- 'What might be done with what I find out?'

This helps you to be clearer about the different types of investigative work you are required to undertake within your medical curriculum. It might be a critical literature review to answer a clinical question or you might undertake a clinical audit, a health service evaluation or some basic research. Clinical audits, health service evaluations and basic research all use similar tools but serve different purposes, as will be explained. Developing good habits in doing and evaluating research is as important for becoming a doctor as mastering clinical skills and knowledge. It's part of developing a professional approach. Medical students are well grounded in the **paradigm** of the natural sciences and this book will show how and why quantitative research is undertaken. However, medical practice also requires doctors to understand social and psychological knowledge, some of which is based in the paradigm of **qualitative research**. These very different types of investigation are also addressed and this chapter orients you to these paradigms.

The differences between the reasons for undertaking basic research and the purposes served by a literature review, health service evaluation, an audit or quality improvement are outlined in this chapter, as is the need for dissemination of research. These aspects are also picked up in more detail in later chapters.

What is research?

'Research' is a word that is applied both loosely to any form of investigation, and also specifically to creating new knowledge. Recently, a prospective medical student said he had *undertaken research* on a topic. However, when the interviewers probed further they found he had read some literature about it and had written up what he'd discovered. As a student you may have an idea that you believe is new but, some months or years later, you find the same idea had already been written about. This shows you are actively engaging with data to make sense of it, but it is also a good reason to conduct a literature review (the topic of Chapter 2) to establish what is already known.

Research aims to derive (sometimes generalisable and new) knowledge from the observation of events. Its purpose may be to:

- test theories and hypotheses or apply models to develop sufficient understanding of relationships in order to predict and so to bring about desired change;

- invent or improve solutions, methodologies and technologies so as to be able to explore new horizons;
- evaluate the success (or otherwise) of interventions (which can be anything from a change in therapeutic practice to organisational structure).

As Figure 1.1 shows, such knowledge may be inductively derived – by repeating observations in a specific context, conclusions about relationships are drawn. This is the kind of thinking a doctor uses when observing signs and symptoms in order to make a diagnosis.

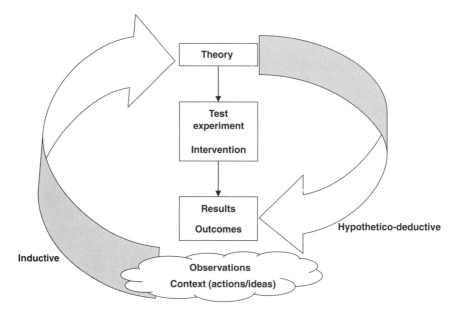

Figure 1.1 Inductive and deductive reasoning in research.

Alternatively researchers draw on models and theories that are then tested against observations – such **deductive reasoning** can never prove the theory or hypothesis but only disprove it (Popper, 1959). Just because you keep seeing events that support your hypothesis, it may be that you have not yet met the event that refutes it. However, if on testing a theory or hypothesis we find it has not been disproved, we gain confidence in it and so continue to use it. Activity 1.1 asks you to apply these concepts about reasoning.

ACTIVITY 1.1 INDUCTIVE OR DEDUCTIVE REASONING?

This week, keep a record of the examples you hear (in lectures or tutorials) or read of **inductive reasoning** and deductive reasoning. Review this daily to see if you can see any patterns emerging (this is induction). Try to explain this (for example, does it relate to who is saying it/the subject matter/the purpose behind the reasoning?), then purposefully seek out situations that will test your hypothesis (or explanation). This is hypothetico-deductive reasoning.

Ways of knowing

In this section we'll first consider what are the bases of knowledge – the epistemo-logical question of 'how do we know' what we claim as knowledge is valid? Why do we believe some things, yet scoff at others? Many who have believed that Santa Claus filled pillow cases know differently now. We are aware that make-believe, opinion, lies, scams and spin are not to be trusted. Yet we accept other knowledge claims.

Reason or logic represents one common-sense way of knowing – internal consist-ency and an absence of logical fallacies or rhetoric can make an argument persuasive. However, what may seem logical may merely reflect social convention. For instance, if you overhear in a conversation, *The baby cried. The mummy picked it up*, it seems logical to think that the baby was picked up by its mother – but nothing you heard states that. You are drawing on social convention for your understanding. The frag-ment of conversation is taken from a lecture of Sacks in the 1960s. He went on to found an influential sociological approach called **conversation analysis**. Abstract concepts may not mean the same to two different people (hence negotiators tend to use them to elicit common ground). An Olympic athlete's statement of being in 'good health' will differ from that of an octogenarian – they have different expecta-tions of their bodies.

Another basis for knowing is to draw on the authority of traditional practice (*it's always been done this way*). Using the wisdom of experts saves time, and indeed the experts may have legitimate claims to their authority. Yet this should not suspend your own critical judgement. Authority may simply reflect power or popularity.

We can also use intuition or revelation that arises from personal experience to 'know' something. This can be a very powerful source of knowledge but it is hard to translate this for others to evaluate. Moreover, it may be just a result of undifferenti-ated other ways of knowing; for example, 'women's intuition' may be nothing more than the close observation of small changes in social behaviour.

We are most likely to trust what we learn from our senses – this is known as empirical knowledge. Bacon's **empiricism** trusted the truth of the senses (we 'know' through sensory perception and observation). This is the basis for the scientific method, and is considered to be objective because other people can repeat the obser-vations and critically review the findings. Yet not everything can be observed directly and our senses can mislead. Moreover, the interpretation of such data is filtered through the researcher's theoretical assumptions. Perception of 'health' through a lens called 'absence of disease' could appear quite differently from a focus on 'resil-ience to disease'.

Why do research?

Medical research saves lives, improves population health and alleviates distress. It is not only basic research – often laboratory-based science – that generates the knowl-edge to do this. Increasingly, the practical benefits of the kinds of observations you can make both as a medical student and later as a doctor are recognised as having the power to make small but crucial changes in practice. For instance, a doctor who noticed the potential for stethoscopes to transmit infection, and put antiseptic solution in a bowl to soak them in next to the sink where staff washed their hands between examining patients, could reduce cross-contamination. It doesn't need a big research study to achieve this desirable outcome: only someone noticing and acting. The intervention is likely to be accepted because of a number of factors:

- hospital-acquired infection is recognised as a concern to be addressed (because of recent outbreaks of preventable disease);
- the principles underlying the proposed intervention are understood and credible;
- the intervention is realistic (it shouldn't undermine current practice nor cost very much to implement).

Can you see how your knowledge about current health policy and what is known to be best practice, as well as your understanding of how to promote change (which means knowing about the local setting of your workplace) can improve patient safety and well-being? Implementing this is the objective of Activity 1.2.

It probably did not take you too much time to reach some useful conclusions.

ACTIVITY 1.2 USING YOUR EYES

The next time you are on a ward, use any time that you have waiting to observe the signage and equipment about hand-hygiene. Where are the signs and equipment placed? Do signs get lost amongst other notices? Does everyone (staff and visitors) heed the instructions? Can you see any improvements that might be made?

There is a trade-off between time and effort and usefulness that is accepted for many types of research, though not all. 'Satisficing' (a management concept meaning data are gathered quickly enough for the results to affect action) is usually good enough for day-to-day research concerning practice. However, to generate believable new knowledge, particularly if it challenges received opinion (the dominant paradigm), requires:

- careful preparation in the selection of the design of the research, and use of the instruments for data collection, to ensure they are **valid** and **reliable**;
- transparency of data recording and analysis;
- careful interpretation of results, including their limitations.

It's the first stage that takes a lot of time.

While it is important to be systematic, to maintain excellent records and to be as rigorous as possible whatever the purpose of your research, if your intention is 'satisficing', it may be that you collect fewer data than is ideal or you 'make do' with proxy measures because they are easier to gather. This is why the success of a vaccination campaign tends to be evaluated not by its effect on disease **outcome** (the incidence of the disease or of complications from becoming infected) but by the easier-to-collect **process measure** of the numbers of children/people immunised. It takes much longer to know how **effective** a campaign was, and in refugee camps or poor countries the health systems may not be able to collect reliable data. In contrast, large-scale and expensive clinical drug trials are required to test the effectiveness of a new therapy. Chapter 10 looks at health service evaluation and explains 'process' and 'outcome'.

There are many reasons why people are drawn to do research. Humans are inquisitive, and often it's simply very engaging and exciting to discover something new or to solve a problem. People explore because they want to make sense of their world. Our world is in constant flux and old knowledge may simply become irrelevant – if not dangerous. Published research can attract, incrementally, new colleagues and fresh ideas. This boost to self-esteem may also be accompanied by the power to influence changes. Solving problems and contributing to social progress have value in themselves. And intellectual property has an economic value. All these are possible reasons for research being considered important today.

Moreover, for reasons of **social accountability**, evaluation research, such as audit and health service evaluation, has become instrumental for organisational learning that feeds into quality improvement. Other reasons why people do research are because a practical problem arises (as with antibiotic resistance) or the possibility for different types of investigation is opened up by new technologies. Inventing spreadsheets, databases and sophisticated statistical packages make it suddenly possible to number-crunch vast quantities of information. Film/digital videos have opened possibilities for qualitative studies because you can now observe people's interactions repeatedly. Mobile phone cameras transmit vivid images of events on the other side of the world to refute claims that *nothing is happening*.

Research is also affected by the zeitgeist of its time and place, and is always grounded in the assumptions and controversies of its discipline. For example, Charles Darwin's and Alfred Wallace's independent discovery that evolution arose from a competitive process of *the survival of the fittest* suited the liberal capitalism of nineteenth-century Britain with its emphasis on market competition. The collection of data for *The Origin of Species* (1859) was influenced by debates voiced among naturalists since the late eighteenth century that all organic species descended from other species (Kass and Kass, 1988). Present-day thinking holds that collaboration between species and organisms is perhaps more important for progress than competition. Symbiosis and networking are keys to success for many life forms. This chimes well with ideas about public–private partnerships and the recognition of the **transactions costs** created by competition in the early twenty-first century. Many think that it is more **efficient** to collaborate in research nowadays.

The varied reasons for doing research are useful to know when you come to appraise a research article critically. Always think about where and when the data were collected, as well as for what purpose. Medical students launching themselves into the unknown may do so for pragmatic reasons (see 'What's the evidence?').

What's the evidence?

Two Cardiff University medical students coding data for a staff project in medical education wrote:

> Being a medical student was a huge advantage to doing this project, not least because being familiar with medical terminology meant that I could understand the transcripts and spot mistakes more easily. As a result of my own experiences of being taught by clinicians I was also able to empathise with the students and make better judgements about why certain actions or phrases occurred. Using qualitative methods to look in fine detail at how clinicians teach (and indeed how students learn) also heightened my awareness of my own professional values and allowed me to learn new skills to become a better teacher myself.... I can also take away valuable theoretical knowledge I have gained relating to medical teaching, and as a result of studying it in such depth I believe I will be a better teacher in the long term.
>
> (Michael Hollifield, personal communication)

> Qualitative research is about discussion and interpretation and as well as learning about coding software, I have learnt how to put forward my ideas and argue my point. In medical education research being a medical student is an advantage as you are an expert as you encounter it every day and you quickly learn to stand your ground to people more senior than you ... Doing research like this is a great thing for a student to be involved in, it does look good on your CV, but also the skills you learn will be used for the rest of your career.
>
> (Blanche Lumb, personal communication)

These students not only gained knowledge themselves but they brought relevant insights to the research. They could interpret the meanings of what they were transcribing and coding (these tasks will be explained later) because they understood the context of the interviews they were listening to.

Healthcare-related research

Medically relevant discovery can happen fortuitously by people who are not clinically qualified. For instance, although the discovery in 1796 of a vaccine to protect against smallpox is attributed to the physician Jenner, relevant knowledge already existed. Lady Mary Wortley Montagu had inoculated her children with material from an infected pustule, and fervently advocated inoculation to members of her family when she returned to England in 1718. She became aware of it in Turkey where her husband was the British Ambassador. The Turks had probably acquired this knowledge from either China or India, where inoculation had been practised since 1000 BCE (Lombard et al., 2007).

However, most medical discoveries have been made through scientific practice. The **hegemony** (dominance) of science as valid knowledge began in Europe in the sixteenth century. Francis Bacon (1561–1626) is credited with first describing the scientific method. He advocated the use of induction of general principles through careful and systematic study of empirical observations. Shortly before his death from pneumonia, Bacon experimented with stuffing a fowl with snow to see if the meat would be preserved – as it was. The scientific method was adopted by both natural and social sciences, but that does not mean that it represents a unified or the only approach, as is explained later.

Underpinning all investigation lie the following factors:

1. a problem to be solved;

2. a desire to find a solution;

3. beliefs and values that determine both what knowledge is considered to be valid (true) and useful and the best paradigm to find out about it;

4. methods and techniques appropriate for finding out;

5. a wish to disseminate the findings appropriately.

In medicine both laboratory-based and practice-based (in clinic and community) research is needed. The early pioneers of allopathic (western) medicine such as the eponymous Dr Hodgkin were able to undertake both (Kass and Kass, 1988). Nowadays, collaboration by teams of specialist experts is more usual. If research is to improve people's health, then discoveries made in the scientific laboratory need to be translated into clinical practice. There is a symbiosis (mutually beneficial relationship) between the resources that basic scientists can develop for clinicians to use and the stimulus for new ideas that clinical observers of the nature and progression of disease may suggest. Basic scientific research into the atom in the twentieth century led to the growth of molecular biology and the development of new materials (both elements and compounds) that changed medical practice. Mapping the genome is resulting in similar advances today. This 'bench-to-bedside' collaboration to the point where the innovation becomes of marketable interest to entrepreneurs (such as pharmaceutical companies or biotechnology industries) is known as **translational research**.

Implementation (or operations) research is another refinement – here the focus is on research that looks at how research outcomes can be put into healthcare practice. It's also known as implementation science or quality improvement research (Sobo *et al.*, 2008). In resource-poor countries the emphasis is on the development of community-based interventions. An example is the introduction by the World Health Organization of insecticide-treated bed nets to control malaria. Many aspects of the local setting will affect uptake, including the delivery of health services, so it is important to know how new products and tools will work in the field. All research conducted overseas needs ethical approval both from the local ethical committee and from the research-ers' academic institution, even though it could be classed as health service evaluation.

Deciding what to research

Research usually starts rather tentatively. Ideas are gradually refined to become specific research questions. With undergraduates it is common for the emphasis in research teaching to be given to mastering the practical skills underpinning research. Students are often involved in other people's studies as a data gatherer or analyst and so aren't actually involved in developing the research question. Nonetheless it is useful to think about where questions come from – not least because it's often something people find daunting.

Where do I start?

If you know what kind of doctor you want to be, you already have a field marked out for you, and locating a project that will further your learning in that field becomes a fruitful effort. If you don't yet know, Activity 1.3 should get you started.

ACTIVITY 1.3

What kind of questions appeal to you? Focus on things that interest you – it's normal for people to gravitate to some topics and reject others as boring. What do you like to do? If you are stuck, think about the following.

One of nanotechnology's purposes is to produce substitutes for natural materials. Would you like to know how to use nanotechnology, or are you more interested to find out how it may affect health inequalities in countries that are dependent on the export of natural resources?

When you go to a meeting or watch television documentaries, what topics enthrall you? Does laboratory work appeal more than talking to strangers, for instance?

Answers to these questions should give you some ideas about where to start looking,

---

To find a question that is possible to answer and which will be interesting and useful, you need to find out about current debates in your field of interest. Reputable journals and public lectures help here. Set time aside weekly to scan the contents, editorials and letters' section of major journals. Do you share the assumptions that underpin them? If not, can you find evidence to challenge them? People (including your supervisor) are another resource to tap into for ideas (Figure 1.2).

Government bodies such as the Audit Commission, the Department of Health and the National Institute for Health Research publish health-related reports. The Department of Health regularly publishes calls for research proposals across a range of issues. These are a rich source of ideas about areas of current concern.

You can build a framework for ideas you garner from these various sources by using mind mapping. Mind mapping is a technique you've probably used for

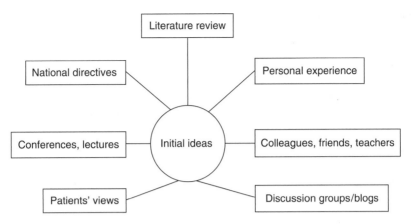

Figure 1.2 Sources of ideas.

essay-writing. It is also useful when generating ideas for research because it allows you to play, explore and link ideas without evaluating them. Pioneered by Tony Buzan, an expert on learning techniques, it frees us from the linear processes associated with reading, writing and logical thinking and so allows us to see ideas spatially (Buzan, 1996). In this way, it becomes possible to make connections between ideas that might otherwise seem completely unrelated (Figure 1.3).

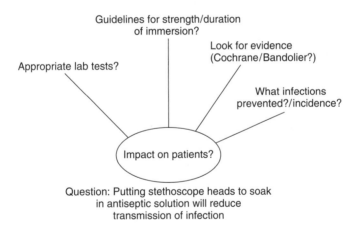

Figure 1.3 Research mind map (initial stage – what to find out).

Not all ideas are researchable. For instance, how much money should be allocated to supporting home care for the elderly is essentially value-driven. It's a political question which will be answered in the context of public opinion and the financial situation. Research could be conducted, however, into how much is actually spent as a proportion of the total healthcare budget and public opinion could then be surveyed as to the response to the findings. You might also research into the impact of spending on the quality of care provided in a number of care homes. This may create an evidence base to persuade politicians to support changes in allocations (or confirm they were acting with political astuteness).

What makes a good question?

Research questions specify the boundaries of the research, what kinds of information will be sought and what types of people or settings will be included. The research question has to be relevant, clear, focused and feasible if the research is to progress successfully. Peter Medawar's book *The Art of the Soluble* (1967) points out the futility of grappling with a problem: if a problem is too ambitious it's the wrong time to try solving it.

The process of refining a research question means clarifying and disentangling various issues associated with the original research idea. You start perhaps with the idea that elderly sick people deserve 'to be treated better' – but what exactly does that mean? Are the drugs they are given making matters worse for them, or are they not being given drugs that could improve matters? If you have an explanation (theory) in mind it's appropriate to form a hypothesis. Otherwise a clear focused question to guide research is best. If explanations suggest themselves as you gather data then you can shift to hypothesis testing. The research question should suggest the study design it is appropriate to adopt. How to develop a clinically useful question is explained in Chapter 2, but to get you thinking about the task, try Activity 1.4.

ACTIVITY 1.4

We live in a demographically ageing society where the prevalence of dementia is rising. People with dementia commonly suffer from agitation and aggression, which cause distress for both relatives and those caring for the patients. Given that many patients with dementia also suffer from painful ailments, it has been suggested that pain may be manifested as agitation by people with impaired cognitive skills.

Construct a feasible research question for a study that might find out how to improve the well-being of patients with dementia.

Research into dementia (as in Activity 1.4) has clear relevance in today's society. Research in nursing homes suggests the prevalence of symptoms of agitation and aggression in people with dementia is over 50 per cent. Antipsychotics are often prescribed for these patients, leading to excess mortality as well as costs (Bannerjee, 2009). 'Can the systematic use of analgesics reduce agitation in residents of nursing homes with moderate to severe dementia?' is a focused question that is feasible to research. Did your answer resemble this at all?

You will be learning to create research questions in Chapter 2, but for now you need to know that what was good about this question is that it is SMART (specific, measurable, achievable, relevant and timely).

Theoretical approaches or paradigms underpinning research

Two very different methodological paradigms (the **positivist** and **interpretivist** approaches) are described in this section. Figure 1.4 shows the relationships between

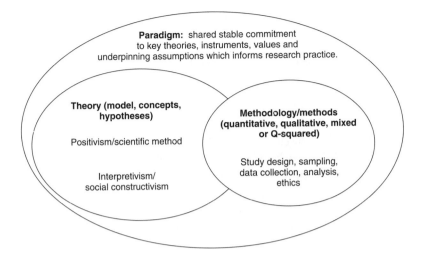

Figure 1.4 The elements of investigation and how they fit together.

the elements of a paradigm. It's these elements that together contribute to the decisions taken when doing research.

Note that the concept of paradigm covers both theory and methodology and also the expected behaviour and values of researchers working within it (Kuhn, 1970). An analogy may help your understanding.

Suppose you've just acquired a horse and want to share the experience with your friends and relatives. There are many ways of achieving that aim, some more practical, quicker or more realistic than others. They include face-to-face meetings, sketching a line drawing, painting an oil picture, taking a photograph, taking an electronic photograph, making a digital video-clip. You choose the digital paradigm rather than the traditional paradigm. But there are still decisions: photo or video? E-mail or upload to Facebook or to YouTube? These design decisions will be influenced by what you want people to see (how handsome the horse is and/or how well he jumps) and your audience (do they have access to the internet? How fast is their broadband connection?). Then you have to decide on your methods: send via your mobile phone or your laptop? Who should see it and by when? Can you block access?

The influence of disciplinary orientation

It is self-evident that in the natural sciences astronomers will draw on a different knowledge base from that relevant to experts in nanotechnology, whilst in the social sciences, economists who model large-scale assumptions contrast with the close empirical inspection of documentary data by some discourse analysts. You don't need to know what these researchers do – it's common sense that scale and topic matter.

Apart from the differences in theory and practice that arise because of what is studied by researchers, there is a fundamental distinction to be made between:

- researchers who focus on how an objectively discoverable reality works (which is the basic premise of the scientific method); and

- those who focus on how people manage to construct shared meaning (reality) through the use of language in social interaction.

Practically, the former (positivism or the scientific method) is associated with quantitative research in both the natural and social sciences and has generated advances in technologies and therapies. The latter (interpretivism or **social constructivism**) is associated with qualitative research and has deepened understanding about how people construct meaning and identity. Non-adherence by adolescents to chelation therapy for thalassaemia (a genetic blood disorder) reflects their wish to assert an independent identity (Atkin and Ahmad, 2000). Healthcare workers who understand this can work with the young person to adjust to the treatment. Such knowledge of people's values and perceptions has a practical application in improving patient care, organisational efficiency or implementing change.

Positivism and interpretivism are two broad paradigms of which you should be aware. Within each approach there are still finer distinctions between schools of thought that only become important when a specific question is posed that is best addressed using a particular theory. For your research at this stage what matters is that you are aware they exist and are different (so you have some understanding about what you may read in the wider research literature).

Using theory helps you know what relevant data to collect. It suggests links that could be fruitful to explore. Underpinning all theories are values and choices. Sometimes if you find ideas difficult to understand it is because you do not share the same view of the world as the person expressing them. Language can impede communication as well as facilitate it.

In hospital-based medicine emphasis has customarily focused on positivist research so you may find it easier to develop research questions that involve quantifying and identifying associations or even causal relationships between variables (Burgoyne *et al.*, 2010; Murdoch-Eaton *et al.*, 2010). **Mixed-method (Q^2)** approaches are increasingly used in complex investigations. We shall look at research methods more closely in Chapter 4.

Research designs

Research may aim to come up either with an explanation or with a description in relation to the topic of interest. Before data collection and analysis can start, the right design is needed to make sure evidence is collected to answer the question as unambiguously as possible. In biomedical research, study designs are classically quantitative: either **controlled** (also called **experimental** or **intervention**) or observational (also called **epidemiological**). They will be discussed in detail below, along with the main types of **qualitative** (or **post-positivist** /interpretivist) research that is also used in clinical research. All have advantages and disadvantages, but controlled designs are the most reliable, and are the gold standard for identifying the cause of an observed **correlation**.

It is customary to distinguish broadly between quantitative and qualitative approaches or paradigms (Figure 1.4). It is the process of measurement used by quantitative research that differentiates the two approaches – qualitative research records and reports in words (and sometimes other media). In contrast, quantitative research counts and measures its subject matter (Table 1.1). It uses numbers both to describe and to analyse. Both paradigms draw on theory whether to:

- test it (hypothetico-deduction);
- to generate new theory (induction);
- to refine conceptual issues (for example, distinguishing between syringes and needles that are unsterile and those that are capable of transmitting HIV could lead you to research the dose of viable HIV needed to infect a person).

Table 1.1 Differences between quantitative and qualitative research

Quantitative research	*Qualitative research*
Deductive approach **Aims** • Tests theory through observations • Oriented to cause and effect • To quantify data and generalise results from a sample to the population of interest	**Inductive approach** **Aims** • Generates theory through observations • Oriented to exploration and discovery • To gain an understanding of underlying reasons and motivations
Procedures • Predetermined design • Analysis follows data collection and coding • Sample: usually a large number of cases representing the population of interest. Randomly selected respondents • Data: structured techniques such as online questionnaires, on-street or telephone interviews • Statistical analysis • Outcome to provide convincing evidence to recommend a course of action	**Procedures** • Emergent design • Merges data collection with ongoing analysis • Sample: usually a small number of non-representative cases. Respondents selected to fulfil a given quota or for theoretical reasons • Data: depends on research but indepth or semistructured interviews common • Constant comparison/thematic analysis • Outcome to develop understanding
Objectivity • Results do not depend on researcher's beliefs • Measurement is stressed • Researcher is detached and distant from data • Standardised protocols are used	**Subjectivity** • Seeks to understand others' motives and perceptions • Emphasises meaning and interpretation • Researcher is the research instrument • Importance of immersion in the data
Universality/generalisability • Emphasises generalisation and replication • Analyses variables • Experimental and statistical controls • Uses large numbers of cases	**Importance of context** • Emphasises depth and detail • Analyses holistic systems • Naturalistic approach • Relies on a few purposively chosen cases

The research question should determine the research study design – although many people often put the cart before the horse. Other factors, such as ethical considerations or logistical feasibility and cost, also affect the selection of a study design. If you want to know if a drug has teratogenic potential it would be unethical to expose pregnant women to it deliberately (in case a baby was born with congenital defects). However, experiments on animal models (such as genetically modified mice) are considered acceptable (though not by everyone). Pregnancy registers are large, **prospective** studies that monitor the exposures that women have when pregnant and then record the outcome of their births. Such studies reveal possible risks of medications (or other exposures) in human pregnancies. A study design is needed that shows the drug causes the effect (the birth defect). A **cross-sectional** survey might show an **association**, but congenital defects are rare events and women will have difficulty recalling the events of the previous nine months, so it would be an unsuitable design.

ACTIVITY 1.5

Google 'thalidomide'. How did the medical establishment discover the consequences of prescribing this drug to pregnant women from 1957? Is it used as a drug these days?

The thalidomide story makes the point that **clinical trials** don't always identify everything at the time. It was clinical reports that alerted the medical establishment quickly to the risk. So research needs to have a wider perspective through public health and data gathering/monitoring. However, routinely collected data cannot be assumed to exist, as the case study below shows. Concerns about breast augmentation Poly Implant Prosthèse (PIP) implants in 2012 highlighted the weaknesses of private medical practices where relevant records and follow-up are not promoted.

Case study: Risks of silicone implants

Throughout the 1980s and 1990s, a number of class actions were brought against Dow Corning, an American manufacturer of silicone breast implants, in several countries, including Australia. Around 400,000 women worldwide were involved in the class action suits.

Claims linked the implants to breast cancer, autoimmune diseases and neurological problems. Such problems led to protracted legal proceedings in a number of countries, significant public controversy and debate, and the filing for bankruptcy by Dow Corning ... In 1999, the US Institute of Medicine's Committee on the Safety of Silicone Breast Implants reported that they had found no evidence for silicone breast implants being associated with any disease. But the Safety of

Silicone Implants report did note a high incidence of more localised complications, including implant rupture, infection and silicone leaking through the nipple or skin.

Significantly, it expressed concern that women who had silicone breast implants had not been informed about potential risks associated to the implants, and that risk of local complications had been understated.

And here we are, three decades later, facing the same issues about breast augmentation but with a different company producing the implants. Again the company is facing bankruptcy, and again, the response to the issue is confused.

We're still unsure about the risks of silicone implants, we have failed to gather any robust or systematic evidence about their safety – even though the Therapeutic Goods Administration (TGA) says that in the last 10 years, around 5000 Australian women have received PIP implants. Because we don't gather data in Australia about who gets what cosmetic procedure, we have little idea of who these women are, who carried out the procedures and whether any of the implants have ruptured. And we have absolutely no idea how many Australian women may have gone abroad, to countries such as Thailand, for their breast implants.

(theconversation.edu.au/pip-breast-implant-controversy-shows-weve-learned-nothing-4896, 2012)

Much of what we know in medicine came about because of meticulous record-keeping by doctors about their patients and this continues to be important. However, undertaking specific research studies enables a more proactive approach to knowledge production.

Quantitative designs

Quantitative study designs, from laboratory-based experiments to the population-based experiments of **randomised controlled trials**, are common in medical research. Counting and scaling are the two processes which create numbers. Counting is done in respect to something which is considered to be important. Noticing how many times a student failed to arrive on time may lead to the discovery that the first bus that can be taken to the early lecture departs too late for students taking it to arrive on time. Scaling is another thing we do routinely, as when parents measure their children's height and say the younger child is growing faster than her sibling. Note there are two scales implicated here: length (tallness) and rate (which includes time).

Comparison between groups is an important aspect of quantitative designs. Studies aimed at quantifying relationships are of two types: descriptive or experimental (Table 1.2). Descriptive studies make no attempt to change behaviour or conditions. Things are measured as they occur.

Table 1.2 Quantitative designs

Experiment	Quasi-experiment	Correlational survey
• Manipulation of independent variable(s) • Random assignment to treatment groups	• Naturally occurring treatment groups • Statistical control of covariate(s)	• Naturally occurring variation in independent variables • Statistical control of covariate(s)
Randomised controlled trials (RCTs) **Cluster** RCTs	Cohort study Case-control study	Cross-sectional survey Ecological study

In quantitative designs it is important to anticipate what variables and relationships are to be analysed – it helps to plan what tables you need in your report so that you make sure you have a large enough sample. In the process of designing an experiment it is important to calculate:

- how large a sample is needed to enable statistical judgements that are accurate and reliable;

- how likely your statistical test will be to detect effects of a given size in a particular situation.

This is known as a **power** analysis. The size of the sample needed is calculated taking into account the frequency with which you expect to find an event happening, and the degree of certainty you wish to establish that your finding could not be happening by chance. In order to get valid results the statistical techniques need to be appropriate for the chosen design. Moreover, it is important that you select an unbiased sample from the population to which you want to generalise your results. Types of samples that can be taken are shown below.

Biased samples	Unbiased samples
Convenience sampling – quick and easy way to obtain data – those people who are in the same class or workplace, for instance	**Simple random sampling** – the sample is chosen randomly from the population using random number tables so that everyone in the population has an equal chance of being selected
Self-selective sampling – population provides information by volunteering their opinions in response to an invitation to comment (as at road show consultations, for instance)	**Stratified random sampling** – the population is divided into groups (strata), then random samples are drawn

Samples might also be taken for theoretical reasons, particularly in qualitative studies. If you wanted to investigate a specific and quite rare disease, the sample would be those patients with that disease whom you had persuaded to form part of your study (purposive or theoretical sampling).

Controlled (experimental/interventional) studies

A **variable** is any entity that can take on different values. An independent variable is one the researcher (or nature) manipulates – the intervention. The dependent variable is the one that is affected by the independent variable (the effect or outcome). Central to the idea of an experiment is that a treatment (or independent) variable can be manipulated and compared with the performance of controls. This makes it a powerful design for explaining cause (independent variable) and effect (the dependent variable). At its most simple, the comparison groups resemble each other in all other variables except for their exposure to the treatment variable. The outcomes (dependent variables) that are measured temporally follow changes in the independent/treatment variable. While experiments (or trials) are straightforward in a laboratory setting, they may pose ethical or logistical problems when applied to communities. In developing countries research may be of minimal relevance to the trial participants' needs but is their only access to healthcare provision (and is time-limited by the trial duration). In epidemiology the **randomised controlled trial** is an experimental design where there is manipulation of the intervention variable and a control group forms the comparison. Watch out for *confounding variables* though!

Observational studies (cohort, case-control and cross-sectional surveys)

Both **cohort** and **case-control studies** can yield information about change over time and thus can make reasonable suggestions about cause (**relative risk** or **odds ratio**). A cohort study starts with the population (cohort) that has been exposed to a risk (believed causal factor) and follows them, usually prospectively, to find out the outcome. Case-control studies start with the outcome (the people with disease) and then question them about exposure. A cross-sectional survey is a snapshot that is particularly useful for establishing the prevalence of disease but only correlations between variables are possible.

Quality of evidence

Each quantitative design differs in the quality of evidence it provides for a cause-and-effect relationship between variables. A well-designed cross-sectional survey or a case-control study can provide evidence for the absence of a relationship if it is not found, but if such a study does reveal a relationship, it is only suggestive evidence of a causal connection. They are thus good starting points to assess the worth of proceeding to designs that are more able to establish a causal relationship. Prospective (cohort) studies, where the cause can be shown to predate the effect, produce more convincing conclusions about cause and effect but they are more difficult and time-consuming to perform. Experimental studies provide the best evidence about how something affects something else, and double-blind randomised controlled trials are the best experiments.

Qualitative designs

Interpretivists (also referred to as post-positivists) are concerned to maintain objectivity even as they seek to build knowledge about values and meaning in people's experience. The techniques of some qualitative designs (such as ethnomethodology, conversation analysis and the development of grounded theory) are rigorously empiricist, being both grounded in data and seeking **generalisable** patterns through a transparent process of coding and analysis that aims to be replicable.

In contrast, other qualitative approaches, such as action research and ethnography, are context-dependent and deliberately use the subjectivity of participation to enrich understanding. Don't worry about the different names given to qualitative designs. It is sufficient at this stage that you recognise these approaches as being qualitative, so that when you read an article the terms have some meaning. When (if) you want to use them there are references in this, and later chapters, to take you further.

Qualitative data are (essentially) information in words about the world, or that aspect of it in which the researcher is interested. Other general terms for this qualitative paradigm are interpretivist/**social constructivist** (Denzin and Lincoln, 1994). Rather than measuring, emphasis is placed on constructing detailed ('thick') description and comparison. Data can be structured or unstructured (not previously coded at the point of data collection as a closed set of analytical categories). Data are collected by asking, watching, participating in events and examining documents from different sources. In the case of **discourse analysis**, close examination of transcripts of conversation is done to uncover tacit rules that help people make sense of what is going on. For instance, how do you know if your friend's remark is joking or serious?

Data gathered within the interpretivist research paradigm are primarily descriptive, although may be also be explanatory. Typically, qualitative designs move from data to concepts (i.e. they are inductive). They address questions about how and why something is happening. By relating events to the wider contexts of time and space they build understanding through elaborating working hypotheses.

Qualitative investigation (particularly **ethnographic research**) involves intensive and ongoing engagement with people functioning in their everyday settings. For example, health services investigators can examine institutional and social practices and processes to identify barriers to change and discover why interventions succeeded or failed as well as what situations and services mean for clients and providers. Ethnography has been used to illuminate the views and experiences of staff working in reproductive health technologies (Ehrich *et al.*, 2010); patient safety (Waring, 2009); and men's experience of erectile dysfunction following treatment for colorectal cancer (Dowswell *et al.*, 2011), for example.

This chapter merely flags up that, within the paradigms of qualitative research, there are further differences in approach that arise because of the origins of the specific tradition, the stance of the investigator and the focus of interest of the research. Figure 1.5 illustrates this by comparing grounded theory with **phenomenology**. To get the best fit between the research question(s) and the study aims, it is necessary to study the

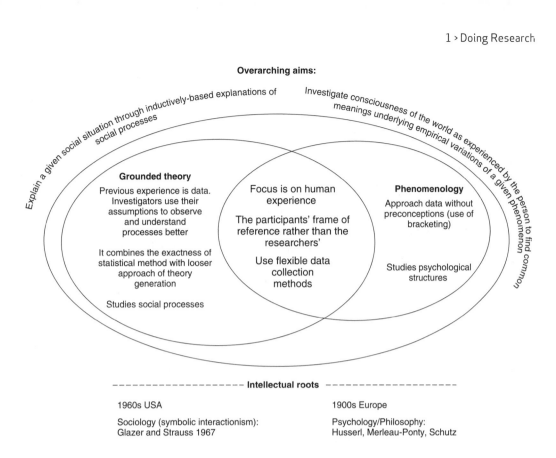

Figure 1.5 A Venn diagram showing the similarities and differences between two common qualitative approaches.

chosen paradigm in detail – its underpinning assumptions as well as its practice and concepts. Denzin and Lincoln's *Handbook of Qualitative Research* (1994) or Bowling and Ebrahim's *Handbook of Health Research Methods* (2009) would be a good place to start.

The research process

Here we signpost what is discussed in later chapters about the process of doing research. Being able to judge the relevance and authority of any given resource for your research is one of the core skills. Chapter 2 will help you with that. Primary sources are the raw material of the research process, such as entries in your laboratory notebooks or completed questionnaires. Journal articles and conference proceedings written by scientists reporting the results of their research are primary documents, as are diaries and autobiographies. Secondary sources (such as textbooks or reviews of research in your topic area) are based on primary sources. Steps in research are as follows:

1. select your topic;

2. choose an appropriate methodology;

3. collect data;

4. analyse data and interpret results;

5. disseminate findings.

Critical thinking

Undisciplined random ideas shared with friends in the pub contrast with the critical thinking required of all graduates. To think critically requires examining all knowledge in the light of the evidence on which it is based, as well as the implications it suggests. Unstated assumptions and values of the author may be revealed in what is (or is not) said and the critical reader is alert to these (just as doctors 'hear' meaning in the patient's hesitations, leading them to question further). You should be aware of lack of clarity in the expression of an argument or deficiencies of logical relationships between propositions. When you examine the quality of evidence you should consider how the research was conducted. That entails examining the methods used and any ethical issues. Ethical considerations concern issues of confidentiality and informed consent (and the anonymising of persons and institutions involved), **beneficence** and **non-maleficence**, explained in Chapter 4. Also, you need to bear in mind the historical context in which the research was undertaken. Wider sociopolitical and cultural factors have a strong bearing on the conduct of research, and may limit the relevance of the application of its findings. This is developed in Chapters 2 and 3.

Table 1.3 presents an overview of the different forms that research in healthcare may take: these are the topics of later chapters.

The overlap between approaches to research with different purposes explains why people often become confused when wondering if ethical approval is needed. Basic research does need ethical approval – but all investigation requires the investigator to behave ethically and to anticipate ethical quandaries throughout the research process.

Chapter summary

In this chapter you have learned that:

- the aim of healthcare and scientific research is to create knowledge that can improve patient care and the contribution that doctors and other health professionals make to well-being;
- different forms of research (laboratory/clinical/population-based; for discovery/explanation/evaluation/development of improved techniques) are associated with different paradigms;
- research is a part of the expectation that clinical staff will continuously update their knowledge, understanding and skills.

Table 1.3 Comparison between research, clinical audit, health service evaluation and quality improvement

	Research	Clinical audit	Health service evaluation	Quality improvement
Purpose of investigation	To generate new knowledge to improve health and well-being – results should be generalisable to the relevant population beyond the specific sample that was investigated	For organisational accountability – results of clinical audit help enforce good clinical practice and produce internal recommendations for any necessary improvements	To produce internal recommendations for local service delivery	To bring about immediate and sustained improvement in clinical care locally
Question considered	It may be tightly specified a priori in the case of an experimental or survey investigation, or may emerge inductively	Does this service reach a predetermined standard of best practice?	Formatively: how can the service be improved (for staff or patients)? Summatively: would another service be more effective or more efficient?	How can the service be improved (for staff or patients)? What organisational (system level) changes are needed to facilitate this?
Methodology	Research should be theoretically driven; can involve patients trying an untested treatment method; patients may be randomly allocated to intervention or control groups	Systematic monitoring of routinely held data and observation of practice. It never involves patients trying new treatment; only routine care is offered and an experimental design is never used	Systematic monitoring of routinely held data may include evaluation using survey questionnaires/focus group interviews. It provides practical information such as costs, benefits, strengths and weaknesses of a service which may involve collecting additional data, but for local use only	This is a multidisciplinary, whole-system approach based on theoretical concepts of total quality management and linked to organisational change. Patients should not be exposed to anything but normal risk
Ethical issues	Research involving NHS staff, patients, their tissue or data, or facilities and equipment requires ethics committee approval	While ethical issues are respected as normal professional practice and it is wise to discuss audit with the trust, formal ethical approval is not needed	While ethical issues are respected as normal professional practice and it is wise to discuss the proposal with the trust, formal ethical approval is not needed	While ethical issues are respected as normal professional practice, formal ethical approval is not needed, although clinical oversight and review are advised

GOING FURTHER

Bowling, A and Ebrahim, S (2009) *Handbook of Health Research Methods: Investigation, measurement and analysis.* Maidenhead: Open University Press.
This is a comprehensive multidisciplinary textbook covering relevant research methods in an accessible way.

Cochrane, AL and Blythe, M (1989) *One Man's Medicine*: *An autobiography of Professor Archie Cochrane.* London: The British Medical Journal.
This highly distinguished medical scientist led an adventurous life. His autobiography is a readable account of his professional development and gives insights into the workings of a scientific mind.

National Institute for Health Research **www.nihr.ac.uk/Pages/default.aspx**
This is a useful portal into NHS resources, reflecting the importance of clinical and applied research.

chapter 2

Doing a Literature Review

Ann K. Allen

Achieving your medical degree

This chapter will help you to begin to meet the following requirements of *Tomorrow's Doctors* (General Medical Council, 2009).

Outcomes 1 – The doctor as a scholar and a scientist

12. Apply scientific method and approaches to medical research.

   (a) Critically appraise the results of relevant diagnostic, prognostic and treatment trials and other qualitative and quantitative studies as reported in the medical and scientific literature.

   (b) Formulate simple relevant research questions in biomedical science, psychosocial science or population science, and design appropriate studies or experiments to address the questions.

   (c) Apply findings from the literature to answer questions raised by specific clinical problems.

Outcomes 2 – The doctor as a practitioner

19. Use information effectively in a medical context.

   (b) Make effective use of computers and other information systems, including storing and retrieving information.

   (d) Access information sources and use the information in relation to patient care, health promotion, giving advice and information to patients, and research and education.

Outcomes 3 – The doctor as a professional

21. Reflect, learn and teach others.

   (b) Establish the foundations for lifelong learning and continuing professional development.

The chapter will also enable you to meet the UK Foundation Curriculum (Academy of Medical Royal Colleges, 2012) requirements for engaging in and understanding research, audit and evaluation.

Chapter overview

After reading this chapter you will be able to:

- explain what a literature review is and why it is conducted;
- explain the difference between a narrative and a systematic literature review;
- outline the benefits to patients and practitioners that result from undertaking literature reviews;
- write a research question;
- use keywords and bibliographic databases to undertake a literature review;
- appraise, and report information so retrieved.

Introduction

We live in 'the information age' – thanks to technological innovation, we are a mouse click away from almost anything we want to know. Our problem becomes not finding information, but sifting through it, trusting it and finding what is most relevant to our study. As a medical student you may sometimes feel overwhelmed by the sheer volume of material that you are expected to make sense of and apply to clinical practice. You'll be 'reading up' on topics all through medical school. There is so much choice it becomes essential to know what you can really trust and that it is up to date.

This chapter shows you how to search the wider literature as well as perform a standard database search to maximise finding:

- the most relevant and up-to-date information;

- information you can use with certainty and so reference in your own work (why you reference is covered in Chapter 8).

After first explaining what a literature review is, the wider context of **evidence-based medicine** (EBM) is outlined. This sets the scene for why and when you do a literature review. How to formulate a clinically relevant question and design a search strategy are described with examples. The need to critically appraise retrieved articles is signposted, with the characteristics of trustworthy evidence being explained. The process of writing up a review through synthesis is contrasted with another type of writing based on literature searches (annotated bibliographies).

Why and how to keep good records is described. Emphasis is placed on keeping a firm hold on the question you are trying to answer for your (and for your future patients' or students') benefit. Anticipating the change (whether personal or professional) that you would like to be the consequence of your investigation will guide you to relevant literature – but you'll also need to judge if what you find is appropriate, credible and timely. In other words, you need to consider the context. The context in which knowledge is produced limits its applicability. For example, drugs tested and shown to work in adult men can behave quite differently in children. Thinking about the context in which it will be applied (does this relate to the essay question?

does this address my research question? will this help my patient?) helps you decide whether findings are applicable, and thus relevant.

Evidence-based medicine

Before we look at how to do a literature review, we'll touch on the wider context that makes it important. This wider context is the increasing acceptance of the principles of EBM since the 1980s, although the term did not become popularised until the 1990s (Darzi, 2008). The term was first coined by a group of clinical epidemiologists based in McMaster University, Hamilton, Canada who criticised the outdatedness of clinical decision-making based on individual experience, calling EBM a new paradigm for medical practice. They wanted doctors to make use of the best and most current clinical research that was published in the literature. EBM involves:

> *tracking down the best external evidence with which to answer our clinical questions. To find out about the accuracy of a diagnostic test, we need to find proper cross sectional studies of patients clinically suspected of harbouring the relevant disorder, not a randomised trial . . . It is when asking questions about therapy that we should try to avoid the non-experimental approaches, since these routinely lead to false positive conclusions about efficacy . . . And if no randomised trial has been carried out for our patient's predicament, we must follow the trail to the next best external evidence and work from there.*
> (Sackett *et al.*, 1996, pp71–2)

EBM may be said to have been fostered by the publication of Archie Cochrane's seminal book *Effectiveness and Efficiency* (1972), which advocated the use of randomised controlled trials (RCTs) to create evidence for the effectiveness of therapeutic practice. The Cochrane Collaboration is an independent, not-for-profit organisation of international volunteers *whose primary aim is to help people make well-informed decisions about healthcare and health policy by preparing and maintaining high quality systematic reviews* **www.thecochranelibrary.com/view/0/AboutTheCochrane-Collaboration.html**

In their everyday practice, doctors are expected to make conscientious, explicit and judicious use of current best evidence. The General Medical Council's (2006) *Good Medical Practice* stipulates this, and that is why EBM is important for your studies as a medical student.

Various sources of evidence exist, including professional experience and expert opinion. Published material is in the public domain so it is open to scrutiny (critical appraisal). You have seen in Chapter 1 how different research paradigms generate different kinds of knowledge. Depending on the issue, many paradigms can contribute to EBM. However, with quantitative methods there is scope for **meta-analysis**. Meta-analysis involves combining the results of several studies that address a set of related research hypotheses so as to estimate the true 'effect size' more powerfully. Many (though not all) **systematic reviews** undertaken by the Cochrane Collaboration undertake such meta-analyses.

Finding and using the most up-to-date evidence is thus a major reason why it is important to do a literature review.

What is a literature review?

There is a difference between a literature review as a process and as a product. The first is what you do to find which articles are relevant for you to read (and which can be safely discarded) for the research you are doing. While the steps given in this chapter are used in that process, the focus is towards undertaking a literature review as an end-product.

Process	Product
This may be more or less focused according to logistics (how much time have you got) and need (what you already know).	These depend on focused and systematic searching towards a defined goal.
To contribute to answering a question (relating to items in the brackets) that may be the subject of:	Narrative review • for an essay; • dissertation/thesis;
• basic research (clinical, scientific, social science and organisational research ...) (Dunne, 2011); • audit (clinical guidelines, previous reports, trust plans, government policy...); • health service evaluation (clinical guidelines, previous reports, trust plans, government policy ...); • a clinical question (a treatment, a prognostic factor, a cause, a screening programme).	• publication as a review article or editorial (Green et al., 2006). Systematic review • Cochrane Collaboration **www.cochrane. org/index.htm** • Campbell Collaboration **www. campbellcollaboration.org/index. shtml**
For any of these, different types of literature may be searched to find information about: • the research setting (contextual factors such as policy, sociocultural and historical characteristics); • the research problem (which may have a number of different aspects depending on the question: risks of arsenic poisoning would look not just at toxicology but also at the epidemiology in occupational groups and/or naturally occurring exposures through bore well water contamination, as in Bangladesh).	Guidelines • National Institute for Health and Clinical Excellence (NICE) **www. nice.org.uk** • Bandolier **www.medicine.ox.ac. uk/bandolier**

In a literature review, you critically evaluate publications about the topic that interests you. You establish what research has been undertaken already by searching, selecting, analysing and then synthesising your findings. 'Synthesising' means that you make your argument through combining the results of your analysis into a coherent whole. It means you bring together the elements of what you've read in order to create something new. This differs from what one often sees described as a 'literature review', which is a list that resembles an annotated bibliography. In this way you build your understanding of what is known (received knowledge) by engaging with it actively.

The point of a literature search is to:

- get all the available information on a subject;
- define and understand prevailing opinions;
- make sense of why people say there is or isn't evidence for something you come across in clinical practice.

For example, most surgeons agree that early feeding of postoperative patients is beneficial, but what is the evidence for this? What we know is that feeding seems to make sense for physiological reasons, but good evidence to support its application could help us to decide 'how soon and on what diet for a patient having undergone what kind of surgery'.

The difference between a narrative and systematic literature review

Medical students learn how to appraise research critically through undertaking ad hoc **narrative reviews**. After critically appraising the strengths and weaknesses of research articles that relate to the question you want to answer, a narrative review synthesises your findings to answer the question you researched objectively. What's often overlooked is the context of the research study (the time, place and personal characteristics that may limit the applicability of the findings, and so determine their relevance). An undergraduate literature review should demonstrate not only library and information skills but *the intellectual capability to justify decisions on the choice of relevant ideas and the ability to assess the value of those ideas in context* (Hart, 1998, p9). Such narrative reviews when published (as editorials, commentaries or reviews) are educational in purpose and may serve to provoke debate about issues of interest to the medical profession. However, they are of limited value for solving a specific clinical problem.

Although in a narrative review you are expected to have searched, recorded and assessed articles systematically, that is not exactly the same as doing a **systematic review**. A systematic review is a formal synthesis of medical research on a particular subject to represent the current state of knowledge about a focused clinical question. Experts rather than medical students create systematic reviews. Teams of researchers volunteer their time to contribute in their area of interest. Where they exist, such reviews form the basis for clinical guidelines. A systematic review uses structured methods to search for and include all (or as much as possible) of the research on the topic. Only relevant, methodologically sound studies are included. Evidence from meta-analysis of RCTs is seen as being the strongest (level Ia or level 1+++), in contrast to that obtained from expert committee reports or authoritative clinical experience (level IV or level 4). The Centre for Evidence-Based Medicine (**www.cebm.net/index. aspx?o=1025**) has posted credible levels of evidence for different kinds of purpose (for instance, to advise about harm from an intervention or about prognosis) (Table 2.1). Systematic reviews can provide an evidence base for clinical standards and guidelines.

Table 2.1 Levels of evidence

Level 1	Evidence from meta-analysis, and systematic reviews of randomised controlled trials (RCTS) and rctS
1++	Very low risk of bias
1+	Low risk of bias
1−	High risk of bias
Level 2	Evidence from case-control studies or cohort studies, including systematic reviews of case-control studies and cohort studies
2++	Very low risk of bias, confounding or chance High probability the relationship is causal
2+	Low risk of bias, confounding or chance Moderate probability the relationship is causal
2−	High risk of bias, confounding or chance Significant risk that the relationship is not causal
Level 3	Evidence from non-analytic studies (case reports, case series)
Level 4	Expert opinion

Source: Nicholson (2011, p245). Reproduced with permission.

The point of emphasising the difference here is because medical students often write in their reports that what they did was 'a systematic review' when what they actually did was review the literature systematically. The correct terms to use in that case are 'narrative review' and 'critical review'. This distinction is elaborated in the following case study.

Case study: The role of the literature review and the shift from ad hoc to systematic reviews

If you read almost any book or journal article that is more than five decades old you'll notice the absence of any systematic literature searching, together with a lack of critical review. Citation seems almost an embellishment to adorn an argument. There were comparatively few publications compared to today but they took time and effort to locate. Hand-searching library shelves and word of mouth were the investigative tools.

Finding a *British Medical Journal* research article on 'Oral treatment of pernicious anaemia: further studies' (Mooney and Heathcote, 1961),

I am struck by a number of contrasts with present-day publications on the same topic. It uses Harvard referencing (rather than the Vancouver style, as is commonplace in clinical publications today). The limited number of references cited by this **case series** span many different journals, the earliest citation being 1948 (when vitamin B_{12} was first isolated), with many published in the early 1950s. At least one relevant American publication was not mentioned (Meyer *et al.*, 1950). I found it through a search on Google Scholar using keywords from the title. Yet the structure of the article follows the standard organisation for a scientific paper (introduction providing a rationale and purpose, methods, results, with tables and figures followed by the discussion). The tone is measured and the outcome of a **controlled experiment** using an oral vitamin B_{12} reported as having favourable outcomes for patients.

In contrast, a more recent systematic review, undertaken for the Cochrane Collaboration (Vidal-Alaball *et al.*, 2005), reported that, with the exception of doctors in Sweden and Canada, intramuscular injections of vitamin B_{12} continued to be used. This systematic review was undertaken 'To assess the effectiveness of oral vitamin B_{12} versus intramuscular vitamin B_{12} for vitamin B_{12} deficiency'. The Cochrane Library, MEDLINE, Embase and Lilacs were searched in early 2005. The bibliographies of all relevant papers identified using this strategy were searched. Additionally the authors contacted authors of relevant studies on vitamin B_{12} research as well as pharmaceutical companies that might know of other published or unpublished studies and ongoing trials. RCTs that examined the use for treatment of oral or intramuscular vitamin B_{12} were selected. Two reviewers independently scrutinised all titles and abstracts identified by the electronic search. Paper copies of all preselected papers were obtained and two researchers independently extracted the data from these studies using piloted data extraction forms. The methodological quality of the included studies was independently assessed by two researchers and disagreements were brought back to the whole group of eight researchers and resolved by consensus.

Two RCTs met the inclusion criteria and the authors concluded:

> The evidence derived from these limited studies suggests that 2000 mcg doses of oral vitamin B_{12} daily and 1000 mcg doses initially daily and thereafter weekly and then monthly may be as effective as intramuscular administration in obtaining short term haematological and neurological responses in vitamin B_{12} deficient patients.

This study (which you can find reported in the Cochrane database) was disseminated through presentations at international conferences.

This case study shows that a systematic review is a major research undertaking, involving a team of researchers and strict protocols. Systematic reviews are possible because of the work of a Scots physician, Archie Cochrane (1909–88). He joined the Medical Research Council's Pneumoconiosis Unit at Llandough Hospital in South Wales. Here he began a series of studies on the health of the population of the Rhonddha Valley, which pioneered the use of RCTs in healthcare policy. He deplored the wastage of resources that the use of non-efficacious therapies created. This advocacy led ultimately to the Cochrane database of systematic reviews, the UK Oxford-based Cochrane Centre, and the international Cochrane Collaboration. Activity 2.1 invites you to explore two websites to find out about available evidence in health and social care.

ACTIVITY 2.1

If you want to find out what research evidence suggests is the best care option for your patient, it is worth looking at two websites that summarise a lot of research:

- The Cochrane Collaboration for health care: **www.cochrane.org/index.htm**;
- Campbell Collaboration for social care (including education and crime and justice): **www.campbellcollaboration.org/index.shtml**

Bookmark both of these websites for future use. Spend about 15 minutes exploring each of them, noting the range of topics they cover and what they report about themselves. Try searching for the answer to a clinical question you are interested in. For instance: could azithromycin be used as a treatment option for a patient with bronchiectasis? (Activity 2.4 picks this up later.)

Opening the Cochrane database gives access to both a summary overview and the detailed report (if you drill down). Detailed reports are informative and may suggest ideas for you to use in searching and reporting your own findings in a narrative review.

Why undertake a literature review?

It's worth reviewing literature for a number of reasons. It saves you time if you find out what has already been reported before you start a new investigation. Finding a recent review article is a godsend if you are unfamiliar with the scope and focus of a new topic, because a good review will identify what is known as well as give useful references to follow up. Often gaps in the evidence are pointed out that you might be interested to research yourself. See Niederstadt and Droste (2010) for an elaboration of these points.

When you start an investigation it is useful to see how others did their research – the study design, the data collection tools as well as the variables studied and the analytic process – and use that to guide your own work. This is why citation and proper referencing are important: you are acknowledging other researchers and your teachers. Through reviewing the literature you will learn about the topic's main concepts, theories and models and how they are applied, as well as the main criticisms that have been lodged.

Another reason for reviewing the literature is to identify the acknowledged authorities in a specialty (by seeing who is cited frequently). 'Citation' is the word used to refer to the acknowledgement given within the text of an argument. Whether as surnames and date (Harvard style of referencing) or numbers (Vancouver style of referencing), they are supported with full bibliographic details in the reference section at the end of a document. Frequent citation is not foolproof though – many research teams, realising that citation was being used both for promotion at work and to secure funding for research, encouraged multiple and rotating authorship as a strategy to secure both. Also some authors are more notorious than others in self-citation.

As an undergraduate you will be asked to write a literature review on a clinical topic which might also form the backdrop for a practical exercise such as an audit or an evaluation of a healthcare service. If you go on to take a research degree such as a Doctor of Philosophy (or an MD) then the literature review serves to show the detailed knowledge and understanding of all relevant research in your topic area (published or not) so that you are able to demonstrate the original contribution of your own research to that field. This is not expected at undergraduate level, but you will be assessed on the rigour with which you search and appraise what you find, and how well you are able to integrate your findings.

People review articles for other reasons than to meet their own knowledge needs. Part of the reason research published in reputable journals is credible is because it has been scrutinised already, as Activity 2.2 shows.

ACTIVITY 2.2

Find and read the open source article by Schroter, S, Black, N, Evans, S, Godlee, F, Osorio, L and Smith, R (2008) What errors do peer reviewers detect, and does training improve their ability to detect them? *Journal of the Royal Society of Medicine*, 101: 507–14. www.ncbi.nlm.nih.gov/pmc/articles/PMC2586872/pdf/507.pdf

---

Articles published in scientific journals are accepted on the basis of peer review. Manuscripts are read by other scientists with relevant expertise, who judge them on the basis of their relevance and the quality of the research – just as you do when you critically appraise a paper (more on this in Chapter 3). It is a way of vouchsafing the trustworthiness of the article. Yet, as the article you've just read in Activity 2.2 shows, the process is not infallible.

On the basis of an experimental study design the authors concluded that editors should not assume that most major flaws will be spotted by reviewers. *British Medical Journal* peer reviewers were randomised to two intervention groups receiving different types of training (face-to-face training or a self-taught package) and a control group. They were all sent the same three papers to review; each paper contained nine major and five minor methodological flaws. The second research question contained in the article's title was also answered: short training packages only marginally improved error detection.

Note how the authors of this paper comment on the limitations of their study. It is worth heeding such points when you read research papers to help you to tune in to potential weaknesses and thus develop your own critical appraisal skills. The explanation that if the article is rejected on the basis of a major flaw in study design, a busy reviewer is not likely to record every flaw seems reasonable. I expect, however, that you probably hope your supervisor, however busy, will nitpick your efforts so as to get things right. Undertaking a literature review to find out what is known thus can teach you also about potential pitfalls in undertaking research.

When do you review literature?

You start your investigations with a literature search for the reasons outlined in the previous section. However, you will probably be searching literature throughout your investigation, even until you have written up your essay or report. This is because as you write/collect and start to analyse data there will be things you want to check, confirm or explain. At the end of a long period of research (say three months for a dissertation) you will want to double-check nothing has appeared in print recently that should be taken into account. You may be certain that your examiners will quickly search the literature and will take note of anything relevant that is missing. The next section takes you through the stages of doing a literature review.

How to do a literature review

Whilst there is a place for browsing current journals (Chapter 1 showed it's a way to discover current debates), it is more **efficient** to search the literature systematically, whether for an essay or the background for a research, an audit or health service evaluation project. If you review literature to answer a clinical question you start by thinking about the patient who prompted the question. The purpose of your investigation will guide what you are looking for. For a clinical audit you would want to find clinical guidelines, but also looking for research papers on the topic can suggest methods and data collection tools that have been validated.

Although in clinical settings most of the questions will relate to the treatment of a condition ('interventions' in EBM), there are many other relevant questions about causation, frequency, diagnosis and prognosis. The PICO (patient/problem, intervention/exposure, comparison and outcome) approach, described below, can yield fruitful questions for all these, though the relevant literature will be different.

Select your topic and devise a working statement

Once the broad topic is selected, narrow it down to a working statement. This forms the basis of your literature search by identifying the topics (potential keywords) you will be using to filter through the databases. The statement does not have to argue for a position or an opinion – that will come from your later reading of what you select.

Examples of working statements, with suggested topics and keywords in square brackets

'Training improves peer reviewers' ability to detect errors' (the hypothesis in Activity 2.2) [training, peer review, error detection]

'The use of, adherence to and opinion towards the current BTS/SIGN guidelines for treatment of asthma in the under 12s, amongst GPs and consultants across six regions in Wales' (audit statement) [BTS/SIGN guidelines, asthma, treatment, children, audit]

'Use of tourniquets in the battlefield' (essay topic) [haemorrhage, exsanguination, injury, trauma, war]

For finding relevant literature you need first to identify the focus of your question. With 'tourniquets in the battlefield' the focus of interest might be: do they save lives – or kill/maim? In what proportions? What could improve matters? Or another focus might be: has the use been adopted in civilian settings?

EBM uses the method of being specific about the patient (or problem), intervention (or exposure), comparison and outcome (PICO) to create relevant and answerable clinical questions. Be specific in defining:

- your patient or problem (age, gender for instance);
- what it is you are studying (a prognostic factor, a treatment, a cause, a screening programme);
- any comparison (another treatment, a **placebo** for example);
- the outcome you are wanting to achieve.

Whatever the purpose of your literature review, breaking the problem into its key components helps to clarify your thinking and to focus the search. So, in an otherwise fit soldier bleeding from bullet injuries and two hours from a field hospital, is it better to apply a tourniquet or use a pressure pad to save his life?

The Cochrane library has a very helpful tutorial for literature searches that includes devising PICO questions. The following activity is drawn from that source but there are many others to practise on: **learntech.physiol.ox.ac.uk/cochrane_tutorial/cochlibd0e4.php**

ACTIVITY 2.3

Mabel is a six-week-old baby at her routine follow-up. She was born prematurely at 35 weeks. You want to tell the parents about her chances of developing hearing problems. What would be a PICO question to frame your literature search?

Activity 2.3 is a question about relative frequency. Using the PICO strategy for this activity results in the very specific question: 'In infants born prematurely (PI), compared with those born at full term (C), what is the subsequent lifetime prevalence of sensory deafness (O)?' This question will help you to find out what to tell the parents about her future risk. These terms (and their **synonyms** – similar words) will be useful keywords for your search:

- P = infants;
- I = premature;
- C = full-term;
- O = sensorial deafness.

Activity 2.4 offers a different example for you to practise with.

ACTIVITY 2.4

You have been sitting in with a consultant in a respiratory clinic where you met a 49-year-old patient who has bronchiectasis. She says that she has suffered from recurrent lower respiratory tract infections in the past year. The consultant tells you that in patients with cystic fibrosis (CF: which this woman does not have), use of a macrolide antibiotic azithromycin has been found to reduce infective exacerbations. You wonder if there is evidence that azithromycin may also be relevant as a treatment option for this patient. Before you proceed to discuss the patient's case with your consultant, you decide to go to primary studies in the literature to help answer your query.

What is the clinical question? _____

_____

Patient/ problem	Intervention	Comparison/ control	Outcome/ effects	Methodology

Question category: Circle one:

Diagnosis	Diagnostic test	Aetiology/harm	Prognosis	Therapy/prevention

Suggested answer:

Clinical question: In patients with non-cystic fibrosis bronchiectasis, can the use of the antibiotic azithromycin reduce the frequency of exacerbations?

PICO:

Patient/ problem	Intervention	Comparison/ control	Outcome/ effects	Methodology
Non-CF bronchiectasis OR Bronchiectasis	Azithromycin	Standard care OR Placebo	Exacerbation rate	Prospective study Retrospective study RCT
AND	AND	AND	AND	

You can see that if you have a number of permutations within a particular PICO category, you'll be using the Boolean operator 'OR' to ensure the terms are all-inclusive within the search. For example, in the first category of patient/problem, the search will include articles which contain either keywords 'non-CF bronchiectasis' or 'bronchiectasis'. Between the PICO categories, however, the Boolean operator 'AND' is automatically assumed as you would want to focus your search for articles that must contain all the terms from each category.

Using the above example, the articles retrieved have to contain keywords from 'patient/problem' category AND 'azithromycin' AND keywords from 'comparison/control' category AND 'exacerbation rate'. You are therefore effectively 'homing in' on the search to include only articles which are the most directly relevant to your clinical question.

The 'methodology' category is used to define further any particular study types you wish to look at.

The question category helps you identify the question type so as to select appropriate **data sets** and study type. For the above question, the question category would be 'therapy/(prevention)'.

The next step in the literature review is the literature search.

Literature search

This section provides information about the use of bibliographic databases and keywords. Recording both the details of your searches (date searched, which database, what keywords used) and the full bibliographic details of relevant articles will prevent you from having to redo your searches later when you compile your sources.

Plan your search strategy – a librarian can help you in identifying databases and keywords.

Bibliographic databases

Abstracts and indexes are tools that make information accessible. Electronic bibliographic databases (such as PubMed) simplify knowledge retrieval, but it is important to be aware that all databases have limitations. This is where the librarian's specialist knowledge is invaluable. Moreover, the more complex the issue, the more unlikely it is that a single search strategy (a protocol defining keywords, databases and inclusion and exclusion criteria at the outset) will suffice, as shown in 'What's the evidence?'

What's the evidence?

In Cochrane reviews of therapeutic interventions, most high quality primary studies could be identified by searching four standard databases – the Cochrane Controlled Trials Register (which contains 79% of studies listed in Cochrane systematic reviews), MEDLINE (69%), Embase (65%), and Science and Social Sciences Citation Indexes (61%). Searching 26 further databases identified only an extra 2.4% of trials. No comparable figures have been published for systematic reviews of complex evidence, which address broad policy questions and synthesise qualitative and quantitative evidence, usually from multiple and disparate sources.

Systematic review of complex evidence cannot rely solely on predefined, protocol driven search strategies, no matter how many databases are searched. Strategies that might seem less efficient (such as browsing library shelves, asking colleagues, pursuing references that look interesting, and simply being alert to serendipitous discovery) may have a better yield per hour spent and are likely to identify important sources that would otherwise be missed. Citation tracking is an important search method for identifying systematic reviews published in obscure journals.

(Greenhalgh and Peacock, 2005. Reproduced with permission.)

You can see that tapping personal networks and serendipity as well as tracking references and citation tracking are useful for finding information. Tracking references means noting references given in the articles you read; citation tracking means tracking who later has cited any useful reference that you read. Nowadays people can post queries to listservs (discussion boards around a particular topic of interest, such as CHILD2015 – Child Healthcare Information and Learning Discussion-group (to register as a member, send an e-mail asking to join: *child2015-admin@dgroups.org*). You can also find articles through search engines such as Google Scholar, although they are not themselves bibliographic databases. Sometimes browsing the library shelves or asking around is very productive, particularly in complex new areas in which people are becoming interested.

Using keywords

Notice how often articles in journals have a list of keywords underneath the abstract. These are chosen by authors to help potential readers find their work in databases through virtual tags. Medical Sub-Headings (MeSH) thesaurus is a controlled vocabulary produced by the US National Library of Medicine. It is used for indexing, cataloguing and searching for biomedical and health-related documents (**www.nlm. nih.gov/mesh**). You can use it to find search terms synonymous with the keywords you identified for your review. Other sources of keywords come from your PICO question, article keywords and sometimes even a thesaurus.

Boolean operators, AND, OR, NOT, can be used when combining two or more search terms. Boolean operators define the relationships between words or groups of words. Counterintuitively, 'AND' narrows your search by retrieving records containing all of the words it separates.

- mouse AND experiment should exclude all articles about breeding pet mice.

'OR' broadens your search and retrieves records containing any of the words it separates.

- mouse OR mice OR rat OR guinea pig (these terms are synonymous in that all are animal models for laboratory experiments)

'NOT' narrows your search and only retrieves records that do not contain the term following it.

- experiment NOT laboratory

( ) groups words or phrases when combining Boolean phrases and shows the order in which relationships should be considered

- (mouse OR mice) AND (gene OR pseudogene)

Search queries containing several operators search in the following order:

( )
NOT
AND
OR

Table 2.2 demonstrates how you can create a search strategy based on your PICO question. There has been much debate in child health about the benefits of early rather than late clamping of the umbilical cord for the preterm infant (fewer than 37 weeks' gestation). The best time to clamp the cord became the subject of a systematic review by Rabe *et al.* (2004).

Table 2.2 Formulating a search strategy using the PICO (patient/problem, intervention/exposure), comparison and outcome) approach

Patient's condition or problem	Intervention	Comparison	Outcome
Preterm **OR** Premature **OR** Infant, premature	Immediate umbilical cord clamping **OR** Synonym 2	Delayed (30 seconds or more) umbilical cord clamping **OR** Synonym 2 **OR**	Requirement for resuscitation **OR** Apgar score at five and ten minutes **OR** Hypothermia during first hour of life on admission or in the labour ward
AND	**AND**	**AND**	

Based on Das *et al*. (2008, p496) and Rabe *et al*. (2004).

As you are doing your literature search it is important to record what you've done. You should list the search terms used, the databases searched, the limits you set yourself and when, as shown in Table 2.3.

Table 2.3 Recording searches pro forma

Database/date of search	Search terms	Limits	Hits	Selected
	Keywords used	*Language and dates and methods are common limits (i.e. it tells the database to ignore anything outside these limits)*	*This gives an idea of how fruitful particular databases are for future searches*	*You should list the bibliographic details of articles to be retrieved in a reference manager such as EndNote or on a separate references pro forma*
Web of Science	Child$ and domestic violence	2000–2006/ English language	276	63
Ovid	Domestic violence/ intimate partner abuse and screening/	2000–2006/ English language/ age group 0–18	170	40

	identification			
Assia	Child$ and domestic violence and screening	2000–2006/English language	2	0
Blackwell synergy	Child$ and domestic violence	2000–2006/social and behavioural sciences	24	0
CINAHL	Domestic violence/ intimate partner abuse and screening/ identification	2000–2006/English language/age group 0–18	83	16
Embase	Domestic violence/ intimate partner abuse and screening/ identification	2000–2006/English language/age group 0–18	50	8

Citation tracking looks for links between authors so as to map out the development of a technique or theory. The strength of this approach to retrieving information is that it is independent of the author's or indexer's choice of keywords. It means locating more recently published articles that cite an older reference. In Activity 2.5 you will practise doing this.

ACTIVITY 2.5

Try this with an article of interest to you that is regarded as seminal (very influential). It must be at least two years old (and perhaps much older – social science articles have a much longer half-life than the biological sciences, where knowledge changes much more rapidly). Find out how many people have cited it, in relation to what research and where the more recent articles have been published. The three original citation indexes (Arts & Humanities, Social Sciences and Science) are available as three separate databases in the ISI Web of Science.

- Log on to ISI Web of Science through your university library.
- Select the 'Cited Reference Search' option.
- Enter the name of your target author in the prescribed format (Surname, initials*) and the year of publication. Note: the asterisk after the initials is necessary.
- Select 'Search'.

Apart from retrieving unexpected articles from different disciplines, this approach allows you to follow up the debate that followed after the original publication. If something is controversial there is generally a flurry of articles either using or refuting the research thesis as other researchers become aware of it.

Selecting, reading and appraising

After retrieving your search results read the abstracts to select those papers that you judge to be:

- methodologically sound (you trust their results);
- sufficiently similar to the context in which you wish to apply it (in terms of the population and socioeconomic and cultural aspects);
- relevant;
- accessible within the timeframe at your disposal. You may also be limited by the language of publication or its cost to view. When you write up your findings you will need to acknowledge these limitations.

This helps you to limit your reading to material that is most useful to you. One of the benefits of belonging to a university is the access it gives you to a wide variety of journals, books and reports.

Once you have read the abstracts you should find either an electronic or paper copy of the articles/books/reports you've selected to read in full. Make sure you've put the full bibliographic source details on anything you have photocopied, and if you have access to a bibliographic database such as EndNote, enter the details on it. Reference managers are software for use in recording bibliographic citations (references), which makes it easy to create a list of articles in the different formats required by publishers or to ensure you've included all relevant details for the references on essays or dissertations. EndNote and Reference Manager are commercial software supported by many universities but there are also open-source web-based ones such as Connotea and Zotero that are free. It's useful to keep any notes in the electronic database for future reference, even if you prefer to use a highlighter pen or to make handwritten notes on the hard copy.

Create a reference pro forma (Table 2.4). If you do this electronically in a database it makes it easy to pull out specific types of study for comparison, but a paper version works well for a small number of references (say 50 or fewer).

Table 2.4 Recording references pro forma

Author/date	Theory/standpoint	Evidence (study design; sample; population, place, time and key results)	Quality of evidence	Comments/ miscellaneous

The following case study gives an example of how to write up a search strategy.

Case study: Writing up the literature search

A literature search was carried out using the databases Ovid MEDLINE and Embase. The term 'male sex workers' was entered into both databases for mapping and the key terms 'prostitution' and 'homosexuality' were combined in both datasets. These were searched concurrently with 'male sex workers' as a keyword. Initially, an attempt was made to combine the outputs of these searches with the term 'health' or 'health services' but this resulted in no hits at all. Therefore, the output of each search was initially screened by title for relevance to the topic and selected articles were then further screened by reading the abstracts. This resulted in 51 articles that were considered to be relevant to the topic under scrutiny.

Database: Ovid MEDLINE(R) ‹1950 to March Week 1 2007›

Search strategy:

---

1 prostitution.mp. or Prostitution/ (3664)
2 male homosexuality.mp. or Homosexuality, Male/ (4464)
3 1 and 2 (141)
4 male sex worker.mp. (39)

Database: EMBASE ‹1980 to 2007 Week 11›

Search strategy:

---

1 prostitution.mp. or PROSTITUTION/ (2687)
2 Homosexuality/ or male homosexuality.mp. (9245)
3 1 and 2 (286)
4 male sex worker.mp. (4)

In the course of reading, other articles were identified that are relevant to the topic under review. These were also obtained and incorporated in the bibliography.

(Sizer, 2007, p7)

Would you agree that there is enough information given in this case study so that you could replicate the search if you were interested? In your critical appraisal you may come across published articles where this cannot be said to be the case. In your own writing up you should try to be explicit about all relevant details. The next section reminds you to critically appraise the articles you've selected – how to do so is dealt with in Chapter 3.

Critical appraisal

After you've conducted the literature search and selected articles that seem relevant, the next step is to critically appraise the material. Critically appraising documentary material enables you to assess the trustworthiness of the evidence that can inform patient care. Researchers from different disciplines conceptualise, explain and investigate differently. They may also use different criteria to evaluate the quality of empirical work. So when you evaluate a paper, think about the disciplinary context in which research was produced. The same words may reflect different concepts. For instance, in political science 'realism' refers to a specific theoretical approach that focuses on state power, while in sociology (another social science), realism is a theory which tries to establish the characteristics of the social structures people inhabit, but also sees them as being produced, reproduced and changed through human agency. What to consider when critically appraising a paper is dealt with in Chapter 3.

Analysis and interpretation of literature

Before you start the process of analysis and interpretation, use the questions posited in the checklist (found in Chapter 3) for the critical appraisal of articles to discard articles that are either not relevant for your purpose, or are methodologically unsound. Chapter 4 gives more information about the hierarchy of evidence and you should use this to rank articles on the references pro forma. The column on your references pro forma for thoughts/comments that occur as you read means this can become the basis for later analysis. Moreover it will provide sufficient context for you to interpret the findings and build a logical argument.

Analysis is a process whereby you break up your data in order to make comparisons between different variables. The question you originally posed (and may have refined) provides a skeleton for your analysis. Read through the comments section of your references pro forma, keeping in mind your original question as you do so. After a while patterns may seem to emerge (or be refuted or confirmed by the absence of rebuttal if you are testing a hypothesis). You may make comparisons on key variables or by theoretical framework or the setting – this will be suggested both by your original question and by growing knowledge of the topic. This progressive focusing is normal so you should allow time for it in your planning.

What you have read may cause you to redefine the research problem, or modify the conceptual framework applied to the problem. Or you may identify methodological shortcomings in a body of research. Where the research produces inconsistent results then plausible explanations may lead to ideas for further research to test emergent hypotheses.

This analysis is not the final stage of your review. The process of the literature review itself will provide a context for understanding what conclusions can logically and feasibly be drawn from the data. Reflecting on this is the crucial stage of interpreting the meaning of what you have found, so that you can argue a plausible case. This part of the process is covered next.

Writing up your review

Remember the aim of a review is to synthesise what is known in order to create knowledge that is more than the sum of its parts. How this is done varies (Tricco *et al.*, 2011). Science and medicine have a standard way to organise research papers including literature reviews using the following structure:

- introduction;

- methods (or methodology for a research thesis);

- results;

- discussion and conclusion.

This is known colloquially as IMRAD. You will have observed this format in the abstracts of published papers, and it is a useful exercise to notice what information appears under each of those headings. Chapter 8 covers how to structure the final report; the following sections address issues relating to integrating the results from a literature search. Other research designs require you to do that, but also to integrate results from other forms of data collection.

Your aim in writing up the results of your literature review is to integrate your findings. That may be done in a variety of ways – but descriptive listing study by study of 'results' is not one of them. The following section shows how to synthesise.

Synthesising the articles

Synthesis involves examining the similarities and differences you found when analysing the articles. Any inconsistencies you find may be explained because different populations were studied or they may reflect different underpinning concepts.

Health inequalities

Today there is little controversy that health inequalities exist (Bartley, 2004). There is wide variation in the health status (morbidity and mortality) of populations at both national and global levels. However, the original materialistic assumptions that this arose from poverty per se (Acheson, 1998; DHSS, 1980) have been challenged by research on relative inequality by others. Marmot (2005), studying British civil servants in Whitehall, and Wilkinson (1996) observed that social positioning and perceived self-efficacy affected not only an individual's sense of well-being, but also measurable indicators of physical health, irrespective of the material conditions of day-to-day life.

The box above not only explains how differing underpinning assumptions about the causes of health inequalities can generate different data but is also an example of synthesising literature. Citations support the argument. Focusing on differences between the conceptual frameworks of the different authors builds an argument that it is possible to explain the existence of health inequalities in rather different ways. This has relevance for action. If a sociological factor, such as material poverty, is the underpinning cause, the policy response is to mitigate it through improved employment or welfare provision. If other factors are also important explanations – psychological ones such as a sense of control or feeling one is of value – then policies preventing workplace bullying and promoting social inclusion become relevant.

Reviews that are not literature reviews

It's so common for students to paraphrase summaries of each article severally (like an annotated bibliography) when what is needed is synthesis that the difference between them needs to be explained. Literature reviews should be organised around ideas. You draw out these ideas as you read the articles you deemed acceptable. Thinking about them in the light of what you set out to discover helps to clarify their significance.

Sometimes people produce annotated bibliographies both for their own use and to help other researchers in their specialty. An annotated bibliography is organised around resources. Full bibliographic details of articles, books and other documents are followed by a brief (about 150 words) descriptive and evaluative paragraph, which is the annotation. This informs a reader about the relevance, accuracy and quality of the source cited. Note how this differs from abstracts in academic articles, which descriptively summarise the content of the article but where it is left to the reader to evaluate the content.

An example of such an annotated bibliography outlining work undertaken in health equity research is Macinko, JA and Starfield, B (2002) Annotated bibliography on equity in health, 1980–2001. *International Journal for Equity in Health* 1(1): 1–20. **www.equityhealthj.com/content/1/1/1**. If you are interested in this research area it's a useful starting point (or you may simply prefer to read a textbook).

Another example is the Influenza Bibliography (**www.nimr.mrc.ac.uk/influenza-bibliography**), maintained since 1971 by the British Medical Research Council National Institute for Medical Research. Every two months it reports on publications drawn from databases such as MEDLINE and Web of Science. Since 1993 it has been available via the internet. The Influenza Bibliography (although not annotated online) is categorised by hyperlinked subspecialty interest. Full bibliographic details are given of materials published since the previous update. See how helpful such a portal might be for someone who wants to keep abreast of current knowledge but who does not have the time to trawl through dozens of journals by doing Activity 2.6.

ACTIVITY 2.6

What information is recorded in the Influenza Bibliography? What other resources and databases are available though this web portal? What are the advantages and drawbacks of such resources?

You can see how it describes what research is being done. Perhaps you explored some of the many different cutting-edge themes in clinical research on this website. Did you think how extremely helpful it is to have such points of access, saving busy practitioners' time in retrieving information? Did you find it difficult to think about the drawbacks? Perhaps you thought about risks relating to sustainability and funding, particularly when topics fall out of political favour. To be really useful such information needs to be current, and archives need to be complete and accessible. Constant software development means archivists face an ongoing challenge to maintain electronic resources.

Chapter summary

The aim of a literature review is to:

- learn about what has already been investigated and reported so as to be able to contribute to knowledge creation in the future;

- be able to critically appraise documentary material so as to assess the trustworthiness of evidence;

- enable retrieval of relevant defensible evidence that can inform patient care.

Systematic reviews provide an evidence base for clinical standards and guidelines. You are expected to be systematic in your approach both to searching for and critically appraising literature because it builds good investigative habits. It also lends credibility to your argument and its conclusions. The use of bibliographic databases and keywords speeds information retrieval, but complex reviews which cross disciplinary boundaries and research designs require more ingenuity than simple adherence to search protocols.

GOING FURTHER

For the Cochrane tutorial on searching literature, go to: **learntech.physiol.ox.ac. uk/cochrane_tutorial/cochlibd0e4.php**

For more information about Medical Sub-Headings (MeSH), go to: **www.nlm.nih. gov/mesh**

Canadian Institute of Health Research (CIHR) **ktclearinghouse.ca**
  This is a repository of Knowledge Translation (KT) resources for individuals who want to learn about the science and practice of KT, and access tools that facilitate their own KT research and practices. This includes materials for learning about EBM and worksheets for critically appraising articles. A tool you might find useful for your portfolio (and personal reflection) is an 'educational prescription', which is a learning prompt for literature review that you can download from **ktclearinghouse. ca/cebm/practise/formulate/eduprescriptions**

Greenhalgh, T (2010) *How to Read a Paper: The basics of evidence-based medicine,* 4th edition. Oxford: Wiley-Blackwell Publishing.
This is a readable, and now classic, book with plenty of examples.

Hart, C (1998) *Doing a Literature Review*. London: SAGE Publications.
Although targeted at postgraduate social scientists, this very readable book has more general application because it gives detailed examples of how to analyse arguments, a map to compare source material as well as showing how to write up a literature review.

chapter 3

Critical Appraisal

Ann K. Allen

Achieving your medical degree

This chapter will help you to begin to meet the following requirements of *Tomorrow's Doctors* (General Medical Council, 2009).

Outcomes 1 – The doctor as a scholar and a scientist

12. Apply scientific method and approaches to medical research.

    (a) Critically appraise the results of relevant diagnostic, prognostic and treatment trials and other qualitative and quantitative studies as reported in the medical and scientific literature.

    (b) Formulate simple relevant research questions in biomedical science, psychosocial science or population science, and design appropriate studies or experiments to address the questions.

    (c) Apply findings from the literature to answer questions raised by specific clinical problems.

Outcomes 2 – The doctor as a practitioner

19. Use information effectively in a medical context.

    (b) Make effective use of computers and other information systems, including storing and retrieving information.

The chapter will also enable you to meet the UK Foundation Curriculum (Academy of Medical Royal Colleges, 2012) requirements for engaging in and understanding research, audit and evaluation.

Chapter overview

After reading this chapter you will be able to:

- explain what is meant by critical appraisal;
- critically appraise literature related to research using different study designs;
- use your knowledge of the practical issues associated with data collection to critically appraise the credibility of research;
- apply these skills to your own research in interpreting your results and writing up your study.

Introduction

In the previous chapters you have seen that critical appraisal of the literature on your research topic is essential. Using the same principles to appraise your own research helps you to get the best out of your research. As well as understanding the strengths and limitations of different methods, you need to approach your own research analysis and interpretation critically in the light of what you actually manage to achieve. As we've noted before, there are always compromises in research – people don't always respond as you would predict and everything takes longer and is harder to achieve than you first thought. But don't let yourself be carried away in your conclusions. Use your understanding to be realistic about what you can really claim to have found in the analysis of your data.

Chapter 2 explained how to undertake a literature search methodically, and how to synthesise the findings to build new knowledge from others' research. You know that relevant articles should be appraised for methodological quality and relevance – and it is this chapter that shows you how to do that. Many of the ideas to be outlined also apply when looking at other forms of information: from routinely collected records to internet blogs to filmed events.

Tools for critical appraisal (essentially checklists of things to look out for) have been developed and this chapter looks at these in greater depth. What is meant by critical appraisal and how to use it is reviewed in the first section. Tips on what to look out for in a variety of study designs used in medical research make up the remainder of the chapter.

What is meant by critical appraisal

After you have conducted a literature search and selected the relevant articles that you want to focus on, the next stage is critical appraisal of the material. This section looks at what should be considered when critically appraising selected articles. You should consider others' ideas whilst critically evaluating their usefulness for your own work. Even if an article turns out not to be relevant, the material may still be useful. It can generate ideas about research design, potential pitfalls or provide a guide to other reference sources.

It is recommended you start with a number of questions in critically appraising an article (**www.patient.co.uk/doctor/Different-Levels-of-Evidence-(Critical-Reading).htm**).

- Is the message important and believable? Do existing knowledge and opinion support it? (Always look for other research, reviews and guidelines on the same topic.)

- Are there any obvious problems with the research? Is it ethical?

- Are the objectives clear? What is the hypothesis or research question being considered?

- How was it funded? Is there any conflict of interest that might threaten the credibility of the published research?

The following box outlines the key criteria you should use when appraising literature.

Checklist to use for the critical appraisal of articles

- Presentation (Is the information clearly communicated? Who is the intended audience? Is it clear what the key message is?)
  Look at language, layout and structure.
- Relevance (Does the information match your needs?)
  Look at the abstract, introduction or overview – what is it mainly about? Does its study population resemble the one you are interested in? In this respect it's important to consider relevant policies (overarching or specific).
- Objectivity (Is the author's position of interest made clear?)
  Look for an introduction or overview – do the writers state their position on the issue? Is the language emotive? Are there hidden, vested interests? Scan the references at the end. You may know enough about the specialty to have an opinion about the standpoints and perspectives of at least some of these authors.
- Method (Is it clear how the data were collected? What type of sample was used? Is the study underpowered (the sample was too small to detect a real difference showing the intervention was effective)? Was the analysis appropriate for the data collected?)
  The methods used should be appropriate and the conclusions supported by the results. See Chapters 1, 4, 5 and 6 for an explanation of these. See also the 'hierarchy of evidence', later in this chapter.
- Provenance (Is it clear where the information has come from?)
  The authors or organisations they work for should be credible sources, as should the publication you accessed. For example, peer-reviewed journals are credible sources. Your medical school library can advise about credible web pages.
- Timeliness (Is it clear when the data were collected?) Note that the publication date can be some years after the data were collected. Also, if the author's argument depends on key publications, check the credibility of those sources, including when their original data were collected. Does the author acknowledge subsequent developments that may be relevant, either conceptually or methodologically? Does the date of the information meet your requirements? Is it obsolete?

You should also reflect on the extent to which an article substantiates or updates other sources you have read, or indeed adds new information. You should explore enough sources to obtain a variety of viewpoints. You will find it useful to construct a pro forma (including a space for the full bibliographic details) so that you can summarise this information as a part of both recording the selection process and the critical analysis that is discussed in the following section. An example is given in Table 3.1 and also in Chapter 2.

Table 3.1 Example of a pro forma to summarise articles for comparison purposes

Bibliographic information	Study type and evidence level	Number of participants	Population characteristics	Outcomes	Results and comments
Aynalem, Smith, Bemis et al. 2006. *Sexually Transmitted Infections*, 82, 439–43	Cross-sectional study Evidence level 2–3	1,351	MSM with a diagnosis of early syphilis who did and did not have sexual encounters at commercial sex venues in Los Angeles, USA N.B.: Biased population as all had syphilis – does not represent the wider population of MSM	Demographic details HIV status Types of sexual practice Condom use Drug use	Men who frequent commercial sex venues are more likely to have STIs, be HIV-positive, have higher numbers of partners, indulge in high-risk sex practices and use drugs/alcohol. Attendance at these venues could be a marker for high-risk sex and STIs.
Bacon, Lum, Hahn et al. 2006. *Sexually Transmitted Diseases*, 33, 228–34	Cross-sectional study Evidence level 3	227	Street-recruited MSM who were intravenous drug abusers in San Francisco, USA N.B.: Biased population as all were drug users	Prevalence of paid sex work HIV status STI history Demographic details Drug behaviour	68% of participants undertook paid sex work. HIV prevalence was 12%. 42% of those HIV-positive were unaware of infection. Condom use was 41%. Higher number of paying male partners was associated with HIV infection.
Weber, Craib, Chan et al. 2001. *International Journal of Epidemiology*, 30, 1449–54	Prospective cohort study Evidence level 2	761	Gay and bisexual men aged 18–30, HIV-negative at time of recruitment, living in Greater Vancouver, Canada	Demographic details Sexual behaviour Sexual coercion Depression scoring Drug use Annual HIV testing	16% reported involvement in sex work. Sex workers were younger, socioeconomically disadvantaged, more likely to have been in jail and to have had non-consensual sex. Drug use was also higher in this group, as was HIV incidence.

MSM, men who have sex with men; HIV, human immunodeficiency virus; STIs, sexually transmitted infections.

Note in Table 3.1 that the graded evidence levels 2–3 in the 'Study type and evidence level' column relate to a subjective assessment of the quality of evidence based on the methods and any flaws observed by the reader (which is a way to start analysing your data as you record it). The numbers represent:

- 1 (high): the described effect is plausible, precisely quantified and not vulnerable to bias;

- 2 (intermediate): the described effect is plausible but is not quantified precisely or may be vulnerable to bias;

- 3 (low): concerns about plausibility or vulnerability to bias severely limit the value of the effect being described and quantified.

For each paper you've chosen to read you should consider how their results (and thus any interpretation) were influenced by its underpinning theoretical assumptions, the study design and the particular context in which the research was undertaken (Chapter 2). In Table 3.1 the analyst has taken account of these factors in assigning a weighting for the quality of evidence – and also in choosing which articles not to use in the final analysis because the context made the findings irrelevant (see the Aynalem *et al.* 2006 citation in Table 3.1).

Hierarchy of evidence

You met the idea of the hierarchy of evidence in Chapter 2 (Table 2.1) but, to remind you, broadly the different levels for obtaining evidence are:

- systematic reviews of randomised controlled trials (RCTs) (experimental designs are 'gold standard');

- analytic studies;
(These aim to quantify the relationship between the effect of an intervention or exposure on an outcome. An analytic study is observational if the researcher investigates exposure and observes outcomes, or experimental where the research actively manipulates a factor by imposing an intervention.)
    - randomised controlled trials;

    - controlled observational studies (cohort studies/case-control studies/analytic cross-sectional);

- descriptive studies
(These don't try to quantify a relationship between the effect of an intervention or exposure on an outcome. They describe what is happening in a population, e.g. the prevalence, incidence or experience of a group. Descriptive studies include case reports, case series and **surveys** (cross-sectional) studies, which measure the frequency of several factors, and hence the size of the problem.)

Many analytic study designs are either not feasible to conduct or not appropriate for answering many questions that as a doctor you might ask, such as: 'what is the likely prognosis for a patient with these characteristics?'

The Centre for Evidence-Based Medicine (CEBM) published a table to identify the different levels of evidence for different types of questions (e.g. prognosis, treatment benefits) in 2009 (updated in September 2011: **www.cebm.net/index. aspx?o=1025**).

- For issues of therapy or treatment, the highest possible level of evidence is a systematic review or meta-analysis of RCTs or an individual RCT.

- For issues of prognosis, the highest possible level of evidence is a systematic review of **inception cohort** studies (persons assembled at a common time early in the development of a specific clinical disorder at the time of diagnosis).

As a medical student you are encouraged to critically appraise research papers because that helps you to learn about the research process (as well as telling you about relevant substantive information). However, when you come to the business of doctoring it is most likely that you will turn to processed information such as clinical guidelines or, if such don't exist, meta-analyses and systematic reviews that have been researched by others. You will appreciate how long the appraisal process takes and these sources are a short cut to good information to inform your practice. Note, however, that the best available published information is only one part of the evidence available to you in taking clinical decisions. The clinical examination, laboratory diagnosis as well as the patient's wishes are all relevant in forming your clinical judgement. However good the external evidence is, it may be inappropriate for an individual patient.

Critically appraising proposals

It is often possible to anticipate problems that may arise in research in the early stages of its design. The following case study of a proposed study will give you an opportunity to practise some critical appraisal skills.

Case study: Proposal to examine psychological problems in students addicted to internet use

Low self-esteem has been linked to addictive behaviours. Craig, S reported that people who hold negative evaluations about themselves use addictive substances to escape or withdraw from their low self-beliefs. Armstrong et al investigated whether low self-esteem was also associated with internet addiction, and found that self-esteem was a good predictor of internet addiction and the amount of time spent online each week.

The study seeks to replicate findings using their operational definition of 'pathological internet use' (PIU internet addiction test) and to extend the findings by investigating the relationship among PIU, self-esteem and affective illness (particularly depression and anxiety, measured by Hospital Anxiety and Depression Scale). University students will be invited (by e-mail, posters displayed on campus and pre-lecture talks) to complete an online questionnaire. They do not have to give contact details, but those who indicate they are willing to participate in a **focus group** interview by completing the questionnaire with their e-mail address will be entered into a randomly selected draw with the opportunity to win a £100 book token.

No potential ethical barriers have been foreseen during this project and the process poses no specific risk to the respondents. We will not gather any personal information about individual respondents nor will we contact carers.

The case study is based on one that was sent to a medical school ethics committee and reflects a number of common errors – which we hope the following three activities will help you to avoid.

ACTIVITY 3.1 SPOT SOME COMMON ERRORS

The first paragraph of the case study is part of the rationale for the research project. What do you think is the research question? What editorial improvements would you advise?

The study intended to describe the prevalence of pathological internet use among university students and whether or not this behaviour was associated with depression, anxiety and low self-esteem.

You probably noticed that the Harvard-style citations omitted the date of publication. Unless there was another 'Craig' publication of the same date, it's usual to give only the surname in the citation. Et al. is an abbreviation so it needs a full stop. If, on looking at the references, the source cited was actually Armstrong and Jones, then et al. should not be used but both surnames should be given.

Taking things a step further (and the date and the article/book title may help you here), you could assess if the citations provide relevant evidence to support the proposed investigation. Here you would need to consider how the authors conducted their research (study design, data collection tools, study population and sampling, for instance) and whether the information given in those papers supports the conclusions that were drawn. And then you would assess if the conclusions could relate to the proposed population to be investigated. For instance, if Craig's research was a small qualitative study of out-of-work Inuit (Eskimo of Canada) and that of Armstrong et al. was based on an internet survey responded to by (according to self-report) middle-aged female divorcees caring for elderly parents, you might feel that the application of their findings is somewhat limited.

Already you may have reasons to doubt the relevance of the sources on which this proposal is based, even though you may feel the study could be relevant and interesting. It might raise in your mind the question, 'If the researchers cannot recognise irrelevant material in what is cited, will they be as casual with the data they collect?'

ACTIVITY 3.2

Do you think the methods are appropriate to meet the study objectives? If you were reading about the research when it was completed and written up, what would you expect to have been taken into account in the interpretation of those results?

Publicity (through posters put up in the Students Union (with permission)/e-mail or texts/call-outs before lectures) will need careful planning. What students are told about the research needs to be thought out carefully. It is vital to stimulate interest if there are to be enough responses. An online cross-sectional survey of student volunteers responding to invitations to participate means consent is implied. Internet addicts may be interested to participate – but if the questionnaire is considered to take too long to complete, the students who do bother to complete it may not be typical of the population of interest (internet addicts who may feel depressed or have low self-esteem). Using this data collection technique is convenient, being both accessible (to a student population) and for processing quantitative data. However, response rates cannot be calculated because the denominator is not known. It is impossible to generalise from a convenience sample.

The questionnaire, even though it draws on ones that are already validated, should still be piloted with students from another similar institution (accessed through friends) to check:

- the questions are understood;
- the responses are meaningful;
- how long it takes to complete.

Using previous study methods (including instruments such as validated questionnaires) is a very good way to learn research skills. It both allows you to focus on collecting and analysing data and means you have something to compare your results with. However, it will not be possible to generalise from the results of this research, and comparisons may thus be difficult to draw.

If focus groups are held as a result of the initial survey it is possible they may yield further useful insights. However, in interpreting any data arising from that it will be important to remember they are self-selected participants and their responses may thus be atypical.

ACTIVITY 3.3

Do you agree there are no ethical issues to be considered in the case study proposal?

The study questionnaire included questions requiring responses to statements such as 'I feel I do not have much to be proud of' or 'I get a sort of frightened feeling as if something awful is going to happen'. If participants are depressed or anxious, how do you think these questions might make them feel? Remember that it is unethical for research to cause harm.

The questionnaire is anonymous – unless individuals want to have their name entered for a prize draw for a £100 book token. For that they have to give their e-mail address. You might reflect whether or not this is an inducement to encourage participation (which is unethical).

We hope critically appraising a research proposal has got you thinking about issues you need to take into account in your own research. Having planned and started your literature search (Chapter 2), you will find it useful to start writing it up while it is fresh in your mind. That helps you to feel that things are moving forward while you spend those hours reading and critiquing the references you found. Similarly, if you are collecting data, start writing and reflecting on its limitations as early as possible. You will come back to what you've written as it needs to be updated, but as you will see in Chapter 8, writing is like that.

This chapter has looked at what critical appraisal entails and has given an overview of the general points to be considered in any critical appraisal. Now the final section of this chapter examines questions as they are applied to research with different study designs.

Appraising different types of study design

This section gives you some ideas about questions to ask of what you are reading with respect to the methodology used. Checklists of relevant questions (for systematic reviews, articles relating to diagnosis or prognosis and RCTs) can be downloaded from CEBM (**www.cebm.net/index.aspx?o=1157**). Your purpose in reading the material is to answer a question that you have formulated (Chapter 2) so an immediate concern will be with the validity and relevance of the results of a study. You judge the worth of what you find on the basis of:

- the results of the study;

- its validity (which will be affected by the processes of selection, measurement (or follow-up for articles on prognosis) and statistical analysis (for quantitative studies);

- its utility – can it help with your decision-making?

In other words, although checklists help you to ensure you address relevant questions, you still need to judge the relevance of what you find for the purpose of your research. *Care is needed to recognise that 'quality of evidence' is not necessarily synonymous with 'strength of recommendation', and vice versa. Judgement is necessary. Only studies seeking outcomes relevant to patients' needs should be used* (**www.cebm. net/index.aspx?o=5513**). However good the evidence is that something works, it still may not be recommended for your patient because of other factors that you are aware of.

Bias and confounding

Bias is any trend in the collection, analysis, interpretation, publication or review of data that can lead to conclusions that are systematically different from the true state of affairs. It's a form of error, but while the effects of randomly distributed errors can be minimised by increasing the size of the study, bias requires attention to the design and implementation of research. It is an issue of study design.

A **confounding variable** is a factor which is significantly associated with both the occurrence of a disease in a population and with one of the causes or determinants, but is not itself a cause. For instance, vegetarians have a lower incidence of obesity than non-vegetarians, but the lower incidence of obesity may be due to the confounding factor that vegetarians tend to be more active as a population than non-vegetarians rather than the lower incidence being due to difference in diet.

Confounding variables can result in erroneous conclusions. Confounding is always a possibility in observational studies – we may not know all the ways in which groups we wish to compare differ. Study design can take this into account through restriction, matching or randomisation. In looking at the effects of smoking on lung cancer we would exclude people whose work exposed them to other sources of smoke. We often match for age, sex and occupational status because these are potentially confounding factors. Randomisation is the only way to deal with unknown confounders. When you are explaining a study result you should search for possible confounding factors.

Appraising systematic reviews

These are regarded as the gold standard of research evidence. Combining the findings of all available relevant research studies with credible methods provides more powerful evidence than could any individual study. However, they can be biased. Those for which no randomised controlled studies were available are particularly prone to bias. Because they are so influential in decision-taking it is vital to critically appraise systematic reviews (Leucht *et al.*, 2009).

Sources of bias for systematic reviews include the following.

- **Selection bias**. Which databases were searched and what were the inclusion criteria? Note what is excluded – could findings differ if research published in French was included, not just the more accessible English articles? For example, in the early 1980s, when HIV/AIDS was emergent in francophone Africa, an inability to read such research limited knowledge. Also if only quantitative studies were reviewed, understanding, relevant for application of findings, will be missing.

- **Publication bias**. Did the authors contact other researchers, and search for unpublished papers? Papers may be unpublished because they do not report any statistically significant findings, but this does not mean that they should be excluded from a systematic review.

- **Heterogeneity**. A major strength of systematic reviews is the meta-analysis of individual study results to produce a combined statistical analysis. The likelihood of the result being due to chance, or to other causes such as inherent differences between studies (known as heterogeneity), can be assessed by the authors of the review. When heterogeneity is identified, a meta-analysis calculation should still be done in order for the review to identify an overall effect or finding, using statistical tests. You should see if this is included in the methodology. If it is not done, then the review is descriptive and so cannot make a convincing case either for or against a change in health professionals' practice.

Appraising randomised controlled trials

RCTs are an epidemiological study design where people are randomly allocated to receive (or not receive) a particular intervention (this could be two different treatments or one treatment and a **placebo**). This experimental study design is used to determine whether an intervention or treatment is more effective than the alternative control (see Chapters 1 and 4). RCTs work well for some types of intervention such as drug trials, but are much more difficult for others and may be ethically inappropriate.

Appraisal of RCTs focuses on the adequacy and appropriateness of:

- recruitment (sample size calculation, selection criteria and randomisation);

- outcome measurements;

- statistical analysis of results.

Bias can creep in at a number of stages.

- Selection and sampling – this can affect the **generalisability** of the findings. What sorts of patient were recruited and from where? Do the inclusion and exclusion criteria make sense?

- Randomisation – were the investigators or respondents aware of their subject/control allocation? Are participants actually assigned randomly?

- Follow-up – sources of bias are *contamination, crossover, compliance, co-intervention, and count (i.e., loss to follow up)* (Attia and Page, 2001, p68).

- Outcomes – were the outcomes that were chosen reasonable? Were all important outcomes considered – and who decided?

- Analysis – this should be done by intention to treat analysis because it preserves the benefit of randomisation.

Appraising cohort studies

Cohort studies are used to investigate causality when an RCT is considered unsuitable, e.g. for ethical reasons. In a cohort study, individuals known to have been exposed to a factor believed to cause disease are followed for a period of time to determine disease incidence at different ages. They are used to study incidence, causation and prognosis. They can measure many factors associated with causation, such as a dose–response relationship or a temporal relationship between exposure and outcome. The main criteria you should look for when appraising cohort studies are:

- the definition and measurement of the exposure (for instance, was there a previously validated questionnaire?). People who suffer from a disease may be more likely to recall an exposure that they think could explain it so recall bias is a problem if there is no independent evidence;

- the selection of subjects (is the sample **representative** of the population to which it relates? Was the sample size large enough to give adequate power? Have possible confounding factors been taken account of? Were some groups unintentionally excluded?). Loss to follow-up is a major source of bias in cohort studies. People who were exposed to the risk factor are more likely to remain in contact with the researchers and this may bias the results;

- the measurement of outcomes (were the outcomes that were chosen reasonable? Were all important outcomes considered – and who decided?). Confounding variables are a source of bias in the analysis of cohort studies;

- make sure that appropriate statistical tests were used in the analysis of results in order to demonstrate any findings suggestive of causality. Cohort studies analyse predictors (risk factors), thereby enabling calculation of **relative risk**. As an observational study it cannot demonstrate causation but the case for a causal relationship is strengthened by:

  - the magnitude of the association;

  - finding it consistently and specifically over time and in different studies;

  - the temporal relationship;

○ if prevention is demonstrated by removing the supposed cause;

○ biological plausibility.

Appraising case-control studies

Case-control studies are used when a disease is relatively rare. They may be used to estimate the **odds ratio** (a measure of risk that approximates to relative risk in a cohort study) which is suggestive of a causal relation. Prospective studies such as a cohort study are more highly rated for giving evidence of a causal relationship than are **retrospective** ones, although the former take many years to perform.

Bias is more likely to arise in retrospective studies. Selection bias occurs in who is selected to be a case or a control (which should ideally come from the same population as the case). The measurement of exposure is another source of bias. Patients with a disease are more likely to recall exposure than those in whom disease is not manifest because they are likely to have thought about what brought about the disease.

'Blinding' (ensuring the person recording information about exposure does not know about the outcome status of the respondent, or vice versa) can overcome observer bias. Standardised data procedures should be used for all respondents.

Appraising qualitative research

Qualitative research does not feature in the hierarchy of evidence, and yet we hope we have shown in Chapter 1 how useful it can be for understanding people's behaviour and perceptions. Qualitative research helps us to understand why people behave as they do, what they value and how they interpret things that happen around them. *Qualitative methods really come into their own when researching uncharted territory – that is where the variables of greatest concern are poorly understood, ill defined and cannot be controlled* (Greenhalgh, 2010, p166). This knowledge is crucial for promoting personal, social or organisational change.

Clinical experience, like qualitative research, is based on observation, reflection and judgement about relevance and how to interpret the significance of what is observed. Clinical practice is enhanced by better knowledge relating to the experiences of patients. There's also increasing recognition of qualitative research being a prerequisite for quantitative research – not only for designing relevant questionnaires but also for generating knowledge that encourages retention in longitudinal studies or identifies constraints to uptake in clinical trials (de Salis *et al.*, 2008). Thus it matters that clinicians are aware of the findings of such research. However, as the next 'What's the evidence?' box shows, the 'checklists' favoured by and used to good effect by EBM can pose problems for researchers wishing to publish their work where it will be read by clinicians, as well as for the critical appraisal of qualitative research.

What's the evidence?

Checklists for improving rigour in qualitative research: a case of the tail wagging the dog?

In medical research the question is no longer whether qualitative methods are valuable but how rigour can be ensured or enhanced. Checklists have played an important role in conferring respectability on qualitative research and in convincing potential sceptics of its thoroughness. They have equipped those unfamiliar with this approach to evaluate or review qualitative work (by providing guidance on crucial questions that need to be asked) and in reminding qualitative researchers of the need for a systematic approach (by providing an aide-mémoire of the various stages involved in research design and data analysis).

Qualitative researchers stress the importance of context but sometimes forget that research itself is carried out against an ever-changing backdrop. Now that it has secured a place in the methodological mainstream, qualitative research is increasingly being influenced by funding and editorial policies. Despite disclaimers by authors that their checklists should be viewed as being 'reflective rather than constitutive of good research,' there is evidence that checklists are sometimes being used prescriptively.

Over the past two years, several researchers have informed me that they must comply with various procedures (such as respondent validation, multiple coding, etc) in order to satisfy the requirements of specific journals where they hope to publish their work. . . . The complex dilemmas in research design that qualitative researchers face with regard to sampling, choice of methods, and approaches to analysis cannot be solved by formulaic responses. If we succumb to the lure of 'one size fits all' solutions, we risk being in a situation where the tail (the checklist) is wagging the dog (the qualitative research).

From reading recent journals and my experience of reviewing journal articles and grant submissions, I find that the five technical fixes currently enjoying the greatest popularity are purposive sampling, grounded theory, multiple coding, triangulation, and respondent validation.

(Barbour, 2001, p1115)

Qualitative researchers need to remain clear about what it is they are researching. The iterative process of modifying data collection and refining hypotheses as knowledge of the topic develops can cloud issues. It is an *in-depth, interpretive task, not a technical procedure* (Greenhalgh, 2010, p167). Taking time out to reflect and review the study findings with colleagues, as well as methodical note-taking about reflections and decisions taken, allows researchers to critically appraise their work and acts as an audit trail.

Because of the necessary variability of qualitative approaches many would see the checklist approach as inappropriate for critically appraising such research (Barbour, 2001; Denzin, 2009; Finlay, 2006). However to appraise an article there are some basic questions you can reasonably ask.

1. Was it appropriate to use a qualitative approach?
   Look at the research question – if it was to gain deeper understanding of a particular clinical issue then it's probably appropriate.

2. Does the research describe an important clinical problem with a clearly formulated question?
   Even though the subject matter of qualitative research (to gain understanding) is fraught with uncertainties at the outset, in order to get anything from the research there must be a clear question to be answered. This should be clear in the rationale: 'Twenty-two elderly residents of a nursing home were interviewed about their dental hygiene' states what was done, but not why, nor why it is important. You should expect to see some relevant background information about the impact of tooth decay on older people's health and the problems associated with maintaining it, as well as the prevalence of dental decay in that population.

3. How were the setting and the subjects chosen?
   While a random sample is essential to generalise to a wider population in quantitative research, in qualitative research it is more usual to select a sample for theoretical reasons (purposive sampling). Respondents are selected because they have particular knowledge or experience, and the researcher will seek to diversify the types of potential experience so as to build insight about the mechanisms at work.
   So if you wanted to understand women's experience of giving birth in hospital you might choose women who had different types of experience (an emergency caesarean section, a late miscarriage, an induced birth, delivered by a medical student). A theoretical sample is not the same as a convenience sample (which is where the first 20 women to enter the nearest labour ward are interviewed because they yield a quick sample). Convenience samples are often used by students (because it's so quick) but, unless the limitations of the approach are recognised, the study is likely to be of little value.

4. What is the researcher's perspective and how is this taken into account in the study?
   You have seen how different research paradigms affect what is asked, observed and recorded. In qualitative research you should expect to see some acknowledgement of the researcher's viewpoint.

5. Are the methods used in data collection described in sufficient detail?
   You have probably noticed that articles reporting qualitative research are considerably longer than those reporting quantitative research. This section is much more discursive because methods are often developed to research a very specific problem. This is in contrast to quantitative research, where a complex diagnostic test can be reduced to a few words and a reference to the paper that originally published it.

6. How did the researcher analyse the data, and what quality controls were implemented?

This should be described in detail, and be appropriate for the theory underpinning it. For instance, if the research is described as grounded theory, look for a 'constant comparison' approach and a search for disconfirming events. Respondent validation is relevant in grounded theory, phenomenology and social action research, but may also be used in other approaches. Multicoding is useful as long as it is done by researchers who understand what they are doing and use it to flesh out conceptual understanding.

The best way to learn how to critically appraise papers is to do it, and ideally share your ideas with others who also have read the paper in a journal club. Many doctors meet at a lunchtime journal club as part of their professional development. Apart from updating themselves in the professional literature, the process of doing critical appraisal can sharpen their thinking about their own research projects. Activity 3.4 asks you to critically appraise two articles.

ACTIVITY 3.4 APPRAISING PAPERS

As you may know already, screening tests should only be used for diseases that are serious but treatable, where early intervention leads to improved outcomes, and for diseases that have a sufficiently high prevalence. The cost of screening should compare favourably with the cost of not screening. The tests themselves must be acceptable to patients and must be reliable and valid.

Read and appraise the following two papers to answer the question: 'Is it effective to screen for domestic abuse?'

Ramsay, J, Richardson, J, Carter, Y, Davidson, L and Feder, G (2002) Should health professionals screen women for domestic violence? Systematic review. *British Medical Journal*, 325: 314–26. www.bmj.com/cgi/reprint/325/7359/314

Yost, N, Bloom, S, McIntyre, D and Leveno, K (2005) A prospective observational study of domestic violence during pregnancy. *Obstetrics and Gynecology*, 106, 61–5. www.greenjournal.org/cgi/reprint/106/1/61

A definitive answer to the question 'Is it effective to screen for domestic abuse?' has not been produced by an appraisal of these two studies. Each has at least one major flaw that draws into question the validity of its conclusion. The systematic review has several possible sources of bias. It did not demonstrate any combined effect through meta-analysis. The interesting findings reported by the cohort study may have been misleading due to confounding, and it also failed to demonstrate relative risk between exposure and outcomes.

Chapter summary

This chapter has:

- described basic editorial and contextual matters to which you need to pay attention when writing up your own research and critically appraising the work of others;

- shown how you might keep records that help with analysis;

- given information on the CEBM, which is a useful source of checklists for different kinds of quantitative reviews (e.g. prognosis, treatment benefits);

- detailed things to consider in critically appraising the most common types of research used in medicine.

GOING FURTHER

Attia, J and Page, J (2001) A graphic framework for teaching critical appraisal of randomised controlled trials. *Evidence Based Medicine*, 6 (3): 68–9.
A detailed account with graphics that explain how to appraise an RCT.

Booth, A (2010) How much searching is enough? Comprehensive versus optimal retrieval for technology assessments. *International Journal of Technology Assessment in Health Care*, 26 (04): 431–5.
This reviews different methods (capture–recapture technique; seeking the disconfirming case; undertaking comparison against a known gold standard; specifying a priori stopping rules and identifying a point of theoretical saturation) that you may find useful for answering a question often asked by students – when to stop!

Dixon, RA, Munro, JF and Silcocks, PB (eds) (1997) *The Evidence Based Medicine Workbook: Critical appraisal for evaluating clinical problem solving*. Oxford: Butterworth-Heinemann.
A very useful and practical workbook that starts from specific clinical problems.

Green, BN, Johnson, CD and Adams, A (2006) Writing narrative literature reviews for peer-reviewed journals: secrets of the trade. *Journal of Chiropractic Medicine*, 5 (3).
A useful 'how to do it' article with examples.

Greenhalgh, T (2010) *How to Read a Paper: The basics of evidence-based medicine*, 4th edition. Oxford: Wiley-Blackwell.
Still the best introduction to critical appraisal of medical papers, and easy to read.

chapter 4

Evaluation and Research Methods
Ann K. Allen

Achieving your medical degree

This chapter will help you to begin to meet the following requirements of *Tomorrow's Doctors* (General Medical Council, 2009).

Outcomes 1 – The doctor as a scholar and a scientist

12. Apply scientific method and approaches to medical research.

Outcomes 3 – The doctor as a professional

21. Reflect, learn and teach others.

   (d) Manage time and prioritise tasks, and work autonomously when necessary and appropriate.

The chapter will also enable you to meet the UK Foundation Curriculum (Academy of Medical Royal Colleges, 2012) requirements for engaging in and understanding research, audit and evaluation.

Chapter overview

After reading this chapter you will be able to:

- construct a scholarly argument for your research rationale;
- explain how the decision you take about your role as an investigator will be affected by the paradigm you've adopted;
- describe the research process;
- outline the limitations of different research designs;
- understand and evaluate what other authors did in their research;
- explain the ethical aspects of doing research.

Introduction

Getting started with research entails thinking about a number of practical matters and this chapter will help you through that process. They involve:

- choosing an appropriate study design method to answer a question;

- selecting which data collection tools to use;

- deciding how to process and analyse the data;

- deciding what it all means and how to present the material so others understand the argument.

These decisions are common to all the different forms of investigation that were described in the first chapter.

The role of an investigator can differ according to the study design (and the purpose of the research). When, and why, participatory approaches to investigation are fruitful will be explained. Political and ethical factors are constantly negotiated in participatory forms of investigation, as you will see. You perhaps already have wondered why some research proposals need to go to an ethics committee but others don't. This chapter will explain why.

This chapter also explains why some types of investigation (such as clinical audit and service evaluation) do not need the formal ethical approval mandatory for conducting original research. Relevant ethical issues (including patient consent) associated with all forms of investigation are signposted and we show how ethical approval is sought for research projects.

Let's start with the basic questions involved in 'finding out more about something':

- 'Why do I want to research this?'

- 'Why have I chosen to do it this way?'

- 'How can my findings be used in clinical practice?'

It's a good idea to research something that really interests you. You may have come across a system on the ward that doesn't work well. You feel strongly about this, want to improve it and you know that you'll need support to bring about change. Therefore, it is incumbent on you to show everyone else (especially the decision makers) that the system you want to improve really doesn't work as well as it could. To convince them, you could pick isolated instances that show that the system has failed, but does this mean that the problem is with the system or with these individual cases? To answer that you need more cases – enough to show that there is a real problem. When you explain your rationale for a study you need to:

- show what the problem is (giving its size or impact, for instance: 'why it matters');

- explain the purpose of the study (to describe, to explain, to see if an intervention works in principle, to try out an intervention . . . or to discover what is yet unknown, for instance);

- give sufficient relevant background for the reader to understand your research question and be able to judge if you've selected the right approach to answer it.

These are the points you would want to make in a scholarly introduction to persuade the reader to continue reading. The case study that follows illustrates this.

Case study: Developing the rationale for an SSC relating to UK refugees

A medical student doing a global health student selected component (SSC) who researched the voucher system available for refugees in the UK decided to interview some refugees and find out whether the vouchers meet their needs. Vouchers are issued weekly and are used to purchase food, clothes and essentials that refugees otherwise could not buy as they are not allowed to work or earn in the UK.

She faced a number of questions: How many people does she need to interview to show that there are real problems with the system? How does she show that the system is at fault? Which part of the system is it that's failing? Does it depend on individual cases? Are interviews the most effective way of showing up the problems? How does she choose whom to interview? What about the voucher providers? Should they put their side of the story across too?

This is what she decided to do: firstly, she reviewed the literature so she could describe how the system works at the moment, including the reason why the voucher system was set up and what it was originally intended to achieve. She then summarised the history of the system, the changes over the years and what has been written about the system, including problems. She set about identifying refugees to interview according to the problems that had already been raised. This could grow into a UK-wide refugee census. But there was really too little time in her SSC to cover the subject comprehensively. Then there was the matter of how much information one interview can yield. Should the same person be interviewed again? Should the cases be followed up?

Time, practicalities and feasibility all dictate how to research a subject. The rationale on which she based her work was formed thus:

There are problems with the system. This has been shown in my literature review and is my justification for undertaking this piece of research. To illustrate the problems I shall interview people who have the problems and show to what extent refugee families from different backgrounds are all affected by the same single prob-

---

lem in the system. As I have decided that my research question is: 'how does the voucher system fail refugees?' rather than 'what are all the faults of the system that fail refugees?' I shall just select a few problems and choose a range of families to interview who have experienced these problems. This means that I can answer my research question precisely and stay faithful to the subject that interests me while undertaking a manageable amount of work. If I wanted to show how large the problem is, I'd count up all the families affected by problems in the system. But that only gives me a number of people (a quantity). It doesn't really give me a measure of how badly affected they are and what they have to do to cope (the quality).

Does choosing a manageable number of families to interview still show that the problem is a significant one? No – only the prevalence of the problem (knowing the quantity so affected) could do that, and this would require a survey of refugees. Then cases could be randomly selected to discuss the nature of the problems that affect them (the quality).

There must be a lot of bias because this is an emotive issue. If I can make my case strongly enough, I can make people see that the system should not remain like this and can show them where they need to make changes and what they need to change to make the system effective. To see whether these changes have solved some of the problems, I ought to wait long enough for more refugees to use the new system, gauge the size of problems again and then interview a sample of refugees who have had these problems and see how they are affected.

This study is essentially an evaluation: she has described the existing structure, how it works (the process) and what the outcomes (and problems) are. By implementing those changes she thinks are necessary and repeating the same research she will have completed what is known as 'action research' (explained later in this chapter).

Your role in research

As a medical student or trainee you are familiar with the idea that the researcher should be objective and neutral so as to 'let the facts speak for themselves'. A different stance towards the research process is that adopted by the investigators you'll hear in the short clip you are going to watch in Activity 4.1. The process of making the video about migrants' lives was intentionally participatory. The researchers have involved themselves alongside the migrants. This type of research has been criticised as being too creative, political or lacking in rigour. Yet such research can be rigorous and scientific. The key is to break every part of the process down to key questions. In the case of the medical student these were:

1. What is the voucher system exactly?

2. Why does it exist?

3. What problem was it designed to address?

4. Does it address these problems satisfactorily?

5. What evidence is there about how it is working?

6. What is the quality of the literature on this that is already available? Is it a fair assessment of the system? Is it an accurate assessment of why the system is not working? Why has it been written? Do non-scientific/personal/political motives cloud the assessment?

7. Based on the assessment, what are the exact problems now? How have they arisen? What are their effects? How might they be resolved/mitigated?

8. Is the problem (and ramifications) big enough to merit research (and then resources that would improve matters for refugees)?

9. How will these changes be implemented?

10. How can we see whether this has improved the system?

Now that every step of an emotive subject is broken down into clear, answerable questions, the research stands up to independent scrutiny.

ACTIVITY 4.1

A two-year Economic & Social Research Council-funded project, Video and Voice in Participatory Research, about the use of video with young people (Kaye Haw and Mark Hadfield) led to the creation of an online resource for researchers: **www. videoandvoice.co.uk/.**

Go to **www.videoandvoice.co.uk/app/case1.html**, case study 1: There is always an agenda.

This video project examined the experiences and perceptions of recent migrants and indigenous young people in Peterborough. A mixed team of community workers, community video makers and researchers undertook the investigation.

Watch the five-minute clip and make notes about what is stated regarding the researcher's role.

The speakers stress that 'transparency' of the process was what was aimed for rather than 'neutrality'. Neutrality is the stance of the investigator as 'objective outsider'. Just as laboratory workers are scrupulous about the cleanliness of materials on their bench, so social scientists working in the positivist (scientific) tradition seek to avoid 'contaminating' the social situation they are studying in order to discover the true reality. In such a situation it is the investigators who set the agenda. It is their decision whom to talk with or observe, when and where. It is their 'purpose' that is paramount.

Yet this stance of being an objective outsider has been challenged. The American sociologist Garfinkel (1967) thought it was important to know how ordinary people made sense of their own lives. He objected to how society was studied in terms of concepts devised by sociologists rather than studying how members of society actually construct the 'seen but unnoticed' rules of everyday life (he called it 'ethnomethodology'). He got his students to break everyday rules – you might try asking in your local market for just a single Brussels sprout and see how the vendor responds!

Breaking an everyday rule shows how we have ideas about what is 'right' or 'normal' in a specific context. We bring preconceptions and expectations into social encounters – even natural scientists have been shown to be subjective in that respect (Kuhn, 1970). Knowledge is always grounded in an historical and organisational context. If we understand those contexts then, even though we may not be certain of the absolute truth of a statement of 'fact', we can still make reasonable assessments about competing claims based on the quality of the evidence and the plausibility of the interpretation.

From the clip you've just seen it's clear that ground rules were agreed at the outset. This didn't stop the young people from exploiting the opportunities offered by the project, however, as you heard. Participants understood what was being handed over and what could be changed and how. The researcher declared: *this is where I am . . . we don't suddenly change the rules*. If the unexpected occurs and rules have to change, then they are discussed. Transparency of process is possible, but neutrality is not. It's the researcher's role to ensure participants understand the difference between *this is my opinion* and *this is what's happening*.

Research that involves health practitioners as co-participants is no less political. With communities you, the investigator, have to facilitate agreement about purpose, practice and ground rules between community members and different agencies with differing agendas and levels of influence. In organisations this process is similar but there is supposedly a common agenda underpinning the investigation. However, different professional groups may hold differing perceptions of the implications of the investigation and their responsibilities. This can obstruct progress if people feel threatened.

As an example, patient safety has become a quality issue in healthcare organisations. Yet in many countries the patient records that could signpost where improvements could be made do not exist. So the World Health Organization (WHO) investigated alternative approaches, as can be seen in 'What's the evidence?'

What's the evidence?

In 2007, after recognizing the difficulties of measuring patient harm (related to unsafe care) in environments with insufficient data collection systems, WHO Patient Safety uncovered from the literature a set of methods to measure harm related to health care and applied adaptations of these methods in various data-poor environments throughout the world to test workload, obstacles (cultural or organizational), relevance, feasibility and acceptability and, when appropriate, validity ... Methods based on direct observations and interviews for measuring the magnitude and nature of adverse events in health care and for defining priorities of action show certain important advantages. The potential benefits of these methods of data collection lie primarily in their capacity to engage the field health-care workers in the research process, thereby contributing to raising their awareness and interest in patient safety, facilitating their training in the identification of harmful incidents and hopefully increasing their commitment towards patient safety. A second advantage is that because these methods are less reliant on existing pre-recorded information, the total cost of collecting the data is in general lower. Moreover, the implementation of some of the methods requires minimal finances, training and competencies – although communication skills are very important, as well as some basic knowledge of qualitative research methods. Finally, a third advantage is that the results of some of the methods are rapidly available, sometimes in real time, enabling a quick and effective feedback loop with the stakeholders of the research process.

(World Health Organization, 2010, pp5–6)

These arguments are persuasive that such investigation must be done constructively. If staff feel 'blamed' by the process they are likely to subvert it rather than assume ownership of it. How such research is introduced, reported and acted on crucially affects the outcome. Research should be seen as a professional commitment, with good practice being encouraged, even if only by its recognition through praise for a job well done.

So if you choose to adopt a more participatory form of research in order to promote change or empower others you need to accept you will have to let go of the 'security blanket' of being the outside expert running the show, and be prepared to negotiate and be transparent in your relationships with others. Action research is a form of qualitative research using this participative approach. It is widely adopted as a research design by people working in the healthcare services and education who are interested in implementing change.

Action research

Action research (also known as participatory research, collaborative inquiry, action learning) differs from other forms of investigation because the people involved become co-investigators. It is particularly suitable for audit and evaluation research because your purpose is to bring about changes that will improve healthcare delivery. People are believed to learn best, and more willingly apply what they have learned, when they do it themselves. Investigation takes place in real-world situations, and aims to solve real problems. Initiating investigators make no attempt to be 'objective' but openly acknowledge their commitment to the other participants. They act as facilitators to nurture local participants to conduct the process themselves.

The key characteristics of action research are as follows.

- It works on, and tries to solve, real practitioner-identified problems of everyday practice.
- It is collaborative and encourages shared involvement.
- It seeks causes to address with solutions.
- The solutions are suggested by the practitioners involved.
- It involves a divergent phase (problem description) and a convergent phase (analysis and evaluation).
- Practitioners decide and plan the intervention themselves.
- Action research puts the planned intervention into practice.
- It evaluates the success of the intervention in solving the identified problem.

It is an approach to problem-solving rather than a defined methodology. It uses various methods, which are generally common to the qualitative research paradigm, and include:

- keeping a research journal;
- document collection and analysis;
- participant observation recordings;
- questionnaire surveys;
- structured and unstructured interviews and focus groups;
- case studies.

Regardless of the study design or the purpose for undertaking research, there are a number of steps to be taken more or less sequentially, as described in the next section.

The research process

Select your topic

Sometimes research is commissioned by policy-makers to support their decision-making, as laid out in a government **White Paper**. Or an unexpected finding from another investigation prompts a wish to understand. Cochrane describes how research on glaucoma in the Rhondda came about through his secretary's mother being treated for the disease. In response to his secretary's concerns he contacted the Senior Registrar and found there was mutual interest in joint research (Cochrane and Blythe, 1989, p197).

Choose an appropriate methodology

Different research methodologies are used because what is considered to be a valid knowledge claim ('evidence') varies both between disciplines and within them. Conceptions about knowledge, available technologies and research practices influence one another and change constantly. Your study design should be described well enough for others to replicate it in the case of quantitative approaches and the more empiricist traditions of qualitative investigation.

For pragmatic reasons, many qualitative studies cannot be specifically replicated although elements of method, participants or findings may be transferable to other contexts. This contrasts with RCTs for example, in which study design, methods and findings are all **generalisable** to a wide range of contexts. Sufficient detail should be given that readers who know something about the substantive areas can judge the soundness of the study. Two investigators in the same place and time might focus on different aspects of what might be considered the same event. One person might address the coping mechanisms that enable people to survive famine, whilst the other may attend more to the interactions between non-governmental organisations, state bureaucrats and the military in constructing a humanitarian response. Readers should be able to read the alternative account and perceive it 'made sense' given the context and detailed information that was supporting the analysis.

Study design

You start by making the following decisions.

- Is the aim to test a hypothesis or to generate a hypothesis?
- Will it be experimental or observational?
- What is to be measured?
- How many and how often?
- At what level (individual or aggregate, for instance)?
- Should cases be prospective or retrospective?

What is chosen will be determined by the question asked, but logistical factors such as available time and other resources are also relevant in practice, as was shown in the case study above of the student SSC. One key decision affecting study design is whether the researcher tries to be a neutral outsider or a participant facilitator and whether people (as patients or as community members) are considered to be:

- 'subjects/respondents/they';

or

- 'partners/co-researchers/we'.

Table 4.1 lists common matters to be considered in a research design. The aim is to collect the right data in the right way so as to be able to answer the original question.

Table 4.1 Matters to consider in research design

Issues	Options
Purpose of study?	Basic research (to describe or to establish causation?), audit, health service evaluation, action research, participatory research
Rationale for study?	Literature review, practical outcomes, develop theory or techniques?
Scope of study?	What is included or excluded and why?
Timing of study	Piloted and phased, duration, exploratory or long-term, currency of findings (importance of wider context of knowledge generation, including socioeconomic factors that may bear on the research)
What is the focus of the research?	Aiming for depth or breadth (case study or survey); what time period? People's behaviour/organisational performance/policy?
What types of data?	Quantitative or qualitative or mixed?
What will be analysed?	Individuals, groups, critical incidents, time periods
Sampling strategy?	Probability, random, quota, purposeful, size, power calculations
Managing data	Record design, data entry, storage, checking, classification, presentation, transcription rules
Analytical approach?	Deductive, inductive, statistical tests
Validity?	Triangulation, multiple data sources, repeated study, comparison with other research
Ethical matters?	Informed consent, confidentiality, data protection
Logistics?	How will access to data (people, events, activities) be arranged? How/when will interviews be recorded or observations made?

In action research the researcher is a participant facilitator. However, the stance of researcher as a neutral outsider is commonly found in medical research, where often an experimental study design is preferred to generate valid knowledge about causation. The experimental research design allows the researcher to control factors that may affect the outcome so that results can be predicted (tested against a hypothesis) and enable valid conclusions to be drawn about the relationships between independent and dependent variables (discussed in Chapter 1). This is done by holding everything except the dependent variable constant (i.e. controlling the situation or context) whilst manipulating (changing) the independent variable to observe the effect on the dependent variable of interest. There are a variety of approaches to this design, as can be seen from Table 4.2.

Table 4.2 Types of quantitative research design

Experimental or longitudinal or repeated measures

- Without a control group
  - Time series
  - Cross-over
- With a control group: randomised controlled trial (RCT)

Observational or descriptive

- Cohort or prospective or longitudinal study
- Case-control or retrospective study
- Cross-sectional survey
- Case study
- Case series

Experimentation is more easily done in the laboratory than in social settings. For choice of medical treatment/intervention, the gold standard is a double-blind randomised controlled trial (RCT) (Figure 4.1).

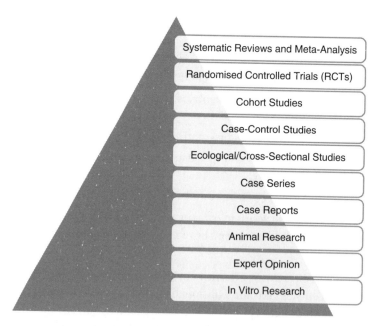

Figure 4.1 The hierarchy of evidence.

Source: Nicholson (2011, p244). Reproduced with permission.

Data collection

Researchers draw on an ever-expanding toolbox for data collection as technologies progress. Interviews (of individuals or different types of groups); participant or non-participant observations; surveys (paper-based or electronic); and laboratory-based tools are all used prospectively. Routinely collected data (such as case notes) have been gathered already, as have records of meetings and other relevant documents, including published and grey literature (unpublished reports and documentary accounts); audio and video recordings, including internet sources such as blogs, are further sources that can be used. These will be discussed in Chapter 5 but common issues relate to access, confidentiality, intellectual property rights (Chapter 8), costs (in terms of resource and time) and the roles of both the researcher(s) and respondents.

Analyse data and interpret results

Chapters 6 and 7 will review this in detail but analysis may be either quantitative, using statistics, or qualitative. Interrelationships between the measured variables and inferences about the meaning of what is observed in the analysis are drawn in the context of the research study.

Dissemination

To make a difference, the findings from well-conducted research should be disseminated: seminar presentations, conferences, publishing either online or in peer-reviewed journals are all ways to make contact both with peers who will scrutinise the work and perhaps themselves take it forward, and with the wider public and policy-makers. Issues relating to this are addressed in Chapter 8.

Ethical and political considerations

Research and evaluation affect people's lives, and so link closely to ethical and political considerations. Often evaluation is used by policy-makers making decisions about a programme or service. Such research is likely to involve change and the exercise of power. But there is no guarantee that the evaluation findings will be acted upon by policy-makers who may have another political agenda, and may ignore or misrepresent the findings.

Building a good working relationship and active involvement of **stakeholders** will help to minimise this risk (WHO, 2010). Ethically, it should be the minimum to expect that research and evaluation are carried out to a high standard and that reporting of problems is done sensitively so as to facilitate any organisational changes to improve services. Some tasks which should be worked through are:

- consideration of the ethical and political factors for all research participants (stakeholders);

- organisation of consent arrangements;

- analysis of risk and benefit;

- talking to clinical and research governance leads about your research/evaluation plan to make arrangements for any appropriate formal ethics approval.

Activity 4.2 shows how these factors were taken into account by a research project to find out potential barriers to uptake of cervical screening in a resource-poor setting in South Africa.

ACTIVITY 4.2

Read Simon, C and Mosavel, M (2010) Community members as recruiters of human subjects: ethical considerations. *American Journal of Bioethics*, 10 (3): 3–11. **www. ncbi.nlm.nih.gov/pmc/articles/PMC3139466/pdf/nihms212939.pdf**

What are the ethical issues surrounding research in which investigators ask community members to engage in research subject recruitment within their own communities? Would they apply to medical students researching the educational (or other) experiences of other medical students?

While the form of sampling you've just read about (known also as 'snowball sampling') is convenient there are problems as Table 4.3 shows.

Table 4.3 Problems with snowball sampling – also known as respondent-driven sampling (RDS)

Type of problem	Example
Bias	1. Initial sample of subjects is not random, but selected on the basis of convenience 2. 'Masking' – certain types of acquaintance of the subject may not be identified for privacy or other reasons 3. Overall sample depends on the size of the network of subjects 4. Subjects tend to recruit other subjects with similar characteristics to themselves
Logistic	1. May be difficult to obtain contact information 2. Subjects may not be willing to provide information
Ethical	It may not be ethical to ask subjects to identify others and provide contact information

Consent

It is a general ethical principle that we do not involve individuals in research without their knowledge, so they can withdraw if they do not wish to participate. This principle is called voluntary informed consent. Decisions on formal consent would depend on the circumstances; for example, presumed consent is made in postal questionnaires when the recipient sends back a completed form. A consent form should be written in clear and understandable language, relevant and focused to what the consent is for. This is underpinned by the researcher's general attitude – respect, empathy and friendliness – which helps participants to develop trust in the process.

Securing informed consent (ensuring people's autonomy by retaining the right to refuse to participate in research) can be problematic. In research where a specific number of participants is needed to demonstrate statistical significance, there may be temptations to overpersuade or abuse a power relationship (such as doctor–patient or teacher–student). There is also the question of people's capability to understand what their participation may entail. Whilst most researchers will assume there is a net benefit from conducting their work, those who participate may not be in a position to benefit from the findings (either because they cannot afford the drug once it comes to market, or it does not address their needs).

Privacy and confidentiality

Privacy is concerned with respecting our right to have control over access to our personal information. Recognising what other people would wish to keep private by putting ourselves in their position can avoid intrusion (which can make others un-cooperative and ultimately will affect the quality of research). Confidentiality stems from privacy and is an agreement about how a person's information will be processed and stored, who may access it and how long it will be kept and destroyed. Anonymity may be ensured by the person's identity not being attached to information about that person. An American study of hand-washing by medical staff, using covert observation, recorded the status of the doctor, trainee or student rather than their names (Haessler *et al.*, 2012). For obvious reasons prior consent of those observed could not be asked, but the research was first cleared with the Director of the Institutional Review Board (as ethics committees are termed in USA). If a formal consent form is used, it should make clear how the above aspects will be addressed. The ease with which data can be transmitted – and mislaid and misused – makes ensuring confidentiality a matter for rigorous attention.

Confidentiality and anonymity cannot always be assumed to be part of evaluation research, due to feasibility issues in certain circumstances. An evaluation of cervical smear techniques in a clinic must be able to identify those people whose skills need updating. Moreover, legitimate praise and publicity for delivering an excellent service could not be given if concerns for confidentiality kept managers uninformed.

Balance of risks and benefits

Apart from the general benefits of research/evaluation discussed so far, there will be risks. These might include social, psychological (or emotional) or even financial risks. Obviously, benefits should outweigh the risks for the stakeholders.

The minimal obligation is that everyone has a realistic appreciation of both the likely risks and benefits when they give their informed consent. People being studied may suffer physical or psychological damage from their participation. Whilst the former may be obvious, detecting the latter is more problematic. In particular, there is the risk of adverse effect happening in drugs trials. For instance, in March 2006 a clinical trial in an independent research unit based at Northwick Park Hospital used healthy volunteers to test an anti-inflammatory drug, TGN1412. Six of them suffered severe reactions, occasioning admission to intensive care (**news.bbc.co.uk/1/hi/ health/4808090.stm**).

What participants may deem acceptable at one time may seem less so to them in the future. Assessing risk is not straightforward: a helpful exercise would be to devise a table of benefits (e.g. list benefits for different stakeholders) versus the risks (pros versus cons).

Researchers should pay attention to people who are vulnerable or at risk. For instance:

- anyone with little power (such as people in prison or hospital, people with learning disabilities);

- anyone who may be damaged by the process or by implementation of the findings (unless the evaluation is to investigate suspected malpractice);

- people in the public eye or who might be placed in the public eye as a result of the evaluation (e.g. victims of crimes);

- children and other vulnerable groups, including those who cannot speak for themselves.

Historically, research has been done 'to' people rather than 'with' them. As researchers we need to be constantly vigilant about power differences in research. Ethical codes make transparent the values and appropriate activities of any professional group. Since Nazi human experimentation in the 1930s and 1940s, close attention has been paid to developing explicit codes of practice for research activity. The **Nuremberg Code** was modified in 1964 by the Declaration of Helsinki when the World Medical Association permitted that research involving children could be carried out provided:

- it would benefit the child population;

- adults would not be an appropriate substitute;

- appropriate consent (or assent where a parent is agreeing to participation on behalf of a child deemed not yet old enough to give informed consent) had been given.

The General Medical Council has a statutory duty to provide ethical guidance for doctors and has detailed material and interactive training materials on its website (**www. gmc-uk.org/**). The UK Medical Research Council (MRC) provides guidelines for MRC-funded research. This is to ensure that high scientific standards are maintained, research is safely conducted, and the wishes and integrity of any involved patients or volunteers are respected (**www.mrc.ac.uk/Ourresearch/Ethicsresearchguidance/ index.htm**). Activity 4.3 helps to place these general ideas into context.

ACTIVITY 4.3

Consider what would be the ethical issues in the case of a project to research either HIV/AIDS transmission or a genetic disorder such as Huntington's disease. Consult **www.gmc-uk.org/guidance/ethical_guidance/5991.asp**.

For example, you might have identified matters relating to confidentiality, informed consent or the possibility of causing harm. Perhaps you thought about psychosocial risks, such as rejection by family; discrimination in employment; and/or restricted or no access to healthcare, insurance and housing. People may misinterpret what they are told about the research. People often apply their own experience with healthcare providers (who prioritise their patient's interests) to the research setting. However, research focuses on scientific and logistical aspects of the investigation as well as taking the interests of the individual participant into account.

It is crucial that as researchers we protect the rights and well-being (**beneficence**) of research participants through informed consent and confidentiality. Note that 'participants' rather than 'subjects' is the noun used. The former signals active engagement of the consenting person (with the right to withdraw respected at any stage) and, associated with this, a respect for that person's autonomy. This also complies with a patient-centred approach to care. Before undertaking any activity participants should have had explained, in a way they can understand:

- the purpose of the research;
- the benefits and risks of participation;
- what participation entails – including the likely time involved;
- who will be sponsoring the research/collecting and analysing data;
- how information will be stored and who will have access to it;
- what measures are in place to protect safety/to make a complaint or ask questions;
- that participation is voluntary;
- whatever they decide will not affect their access to future care.

Protecting confidentiality in the context of research entails ensuring anonymity and privacy at all stages of the research, including after the findings have been published (Broom *et al.*, 2009).

Who is involved in ethical consent?

Medical schools and universities have their own arrangements for giving ethical approval to student and staff research projects, especially those involving education. It is useful, however, when you work with someone else on a health improvement project or clinical trial that involves patients for you to be aware of the bigger picture in the health service.

Local research ethics committees (LRECs)

LRECs evaluate all research proposals involving the use of patients or NHS staff to ensure that they meet the ethical principles discussed above, and that the research will be legal within the Human Rights Act 1998. They are responsible for assessing proposals for research from all health disciplines on a timetabled schedule. If the research involves a number of locations, the researcher may apply to a regionally based committee called a multicentre research ethics committee (MREC) instead.

Submitting a proposal to an LREC usually involves filling in a standardised application form that will ask questions about the following:

- the scientific merit, which includes:
  - aims of the research;
  - potential benefits to patients and/or expected contribution to knowledge;
  - research design;
  - sampling methods;
  - setting and timescale;
- potential ethical issues, including:
  - any procedures, interventions or treatments;
  - any potential risks;
  - procedures for giving information;
  - consent procedures;
  - any payments or reimbursements to participants;
  - indemnity;
  - provisions for data storage.

Ensuring that patients/clients and healthcare staff are not 'over-researched' is another LREC concern. A proposal may be refused simply because many other activities are taking place in the same area. Another common reason for refusal is that the research proposal is not sufficiently explicit about the reasons behind decisions and processes in the research design.

ACTIVITY 4.4

Find out the date of the next ethical committee meeting for approval of student research projects in your medical school. How often does it meet, and how late before a meeting is a proposal accepted? What forms need to be completed and what information is required? Estimate how much time this process will take, and use this to inform yourself when to start planning a research project.

Participants must not be offered financial inducements to participate. LRECs will usually require that participants are reimbursed only for essential expenses such as travel. It is necessary to find out when the LREC meets, and the form a proposal takes. Universities also have research ethics committees to review research that does not require LREC approval (Table 4.4). Securing ethical approval is a lengthy process that requires considerable planning and multiple copies of proposals.

Table 4.4 An example of a project not needing local research ethics committee approval

Your research project involves:	*Yes*	*No*
1 Patients and users of the NHS. This is intended to mean all potential research participants recruited by virtue of the patient's or user's past or present treatment by, or use of, the NHS. It includes NHS patients treated under contracts with private-sector institutions		No
2 Individuals identified as potential research participants because of their status as relatives or carers of patients and users of the NHS, as defined in 1		No
3 Access to data, organs or other bodily material of past and present NHS patients		No
4 Fetal material and IVF involving NHS patients		No
5 The recently dead in NHS premises		No

IVF, in vitro fertilisation.

If you have answered yes to any of the above, then your project is not of relevance to the medical school research ethics committee and, under National Research Ethics Service regulations, ethical approval must instead be sought from the appropriate NHS local/multicentre research ethics committee.

Chapter summary

- Focus on what interests you, whatever the investigation. If you are assigned a task, find the aspects that give you pleasure and a sense of achievement.

- Research questions must be relevant, clear, focused and feasible.

- The research question should determine study design and the population studied.

- Two commonly used designs in healthcare research are action research (qualitative) and experimental (quantitative).

- Ethical issues of informed consent, confidentiality and benefit outweighing cost are paramount regardless of the purpose of the research.

The stance of the researcher, as much as the research question, affects the extent to which service users are involved in the clinical research process (whether they are also involved in its design, for instance) and how multidisciplinary is the clinical team. Any form of action research will include all stakeholders at all stages, for instance, whereas positivist researchers seek to preserve objectivity by keeping control at every stage.

Haw, K and Hadfield, M (2011) *Video in Social Science Research*. London: Routledge.
Not a 'how to' book but a very readable introduction to what you need to think about if you plan to use video in research.

Haw, K and Hadfield, M (undated) *Video and Voice in Participatory Research*. **www.videoandvoice.co.uk/**.
Differing Approaches *looks at the use of video in a wide range of projects and is based on the work of six different researchers and groups. Each case study is a short five-minute discussion by these researchers about their approaches and the issues they faced in working in this way. Browse for a wide range of approaches and comments on the ethics of participatory research.*

The following websites are invaluable starting points for questions you may have about ethics:

Medical Research Council **www.mrc.ac.uk/Ourresearch/Ethicsresearchguidance/index.htm**.

NRES Ethics Consultation E-Group (April 2007) – *differentiating audit, service evaluation and research. NHS Direct website:* **www.nhsdirect.nhs.uk/Commissioners/ResearchServiceEvaluationClinicalAudit/ServiceEvaluation**.

chapter 5

Data Collection and Information Gathering
Ann K. Allen

Achieving your medical degree

This chapter will help you to begin to meet the following requirements of *Tomorrow's Doctors* (General Medical Council, 2009).

Outcomes 1 – The doctor as a scholar and a scientist

12. Apply scientific method and approaches to medical research.

The chapter will also enable you to meet the UK Foundation Curriculum (Academy of Medical Royal Colleges, 2012) requirements for engaging in and understanding research, audit and evaluation.

Chapter overview

After reading this chapter you will be able to:

- identify and make use of a wide range of appropriate sources of information;
- explain factors that affect data collection from a variety of sources;
- explain how different types of data are collected and how the data collection methods are influenced by the research paradigm you use as well as logistical matters;
- explain how to verify the data you are collecting;
- decide what data you need for your particular research and how to access it;
- describe how to store and dispose of your data.

How to analyse the data you have collected is explained in Chapter 6.

Introduction

This chapter describes tools for collecting data that will answer your research question. These tools boil down to asking questions, observing behaviour and retrieving relevant documents (ranging from patient case notes and clinical guidelines to policy White Papers). These will be covered in later sections after we have looked at how to get access. First there are a few important concepts to get your head around: data, information and tools.

The difference between 'data' and 'information' is that data are raw: data are what is collected (numbers, images, responses, activities) while information is data that has been processed and given meaning by making relational connections. A patient's temperature is data; entered on a chart and compared with previous recordings and in the light of results from other diagnostic tests it becomes information that might mean the patient is recovering or not and helps us decide on action. This chapter will focus on data collection rather than information because knowing the problems that can arise in collecting raw data helps in critically appraising the extent to which results are reasonably interpreted in both your own and others' research.

What previous researchers have found to be informative sources of data (and how they overcame any problems with them) can be discovered through a literature review (see Chapter 2). What this chapter refers to as tools are also called 'methods' or 'instruments'. Tools that are standardised can be used for comparison and enumeration in quantitative research, but it is a mistake to think that it is the tool that defines the study design as being quantitative or qualitative (rather, it is the other way around – tools are modified by their purpose). Interviews can be used to collect data in experiments as well as in action research; standardised observation schedules may be used in both quantitative and qualitative research studies. Transcripts of interviews can be treated as data about an underlying reality or may be analysed in terms of how such 'reality' is constructed. The study's design and the data collection tools are influenced by the theoretical paradigm of the researcher and the purpose for data collection.

This chapter examines the practicalities of the tools used to investigate. Your research question should guide choices about study design (quantitative, qualitative or mixed-method), data collection, **protocols** and tools (laboratory notebooks, interview schedules, field notes, observation guides). There are a number of practical matters to be considered before data can be collected, which were flagged in Chapter 4, Table 4.1. Before you can start collecting data, you need to gain access to the relevant people, organisation or documents, and the tool selected may be chosen because it is the most feasible one rather then the ideal one.

Access

Time and frequent meetings to build trust may be needed to find out about some things. With sensitive issues such as strategies to cope with bereavement or examination failure, people reveal themselves slowly. Events that happen rarely may have to be asked about rather than observed (though there may be supportive material evidence in the form of film or photographs or other memorabilia). However, other factors besides appropriateness come into play: as you have seen from Chapter 4, constraints (of resource and time) will have influenced the study design. The investigator's stance – whether to be an objective observer, or a facilitative mentor of others' empowerment through participatory research – is also important (Chapter 4). Gaining access to data raises general issues that tie closely to requirements for anonymity and confidentiality when recruitment is by community members (Simon and Mosavel, 2010).

Any study involving people (as patients, carers, the public or other stakeholders) means you have to think early on about how to recruit them. The design of information sheets and consent forms as well as the strategy used to approach people flow from these initial thoughts, as we will see later. There may be particular 'gatekeepers' who need to be approached first (people who control access to participants: for instance, parents and teachers in the case of research with children). You need to make sure that you involve those who will help you approach the people you will study and that you have their trust, cooperation and consent. You should discuss all your plans with your supervisor and be proactive in designing your methods so that you know early on exactly what your supervisor needs to help you with.

Organisations conducting surveys (for instance, of health staff) need a **sampling frame** (a comprehensive list of names and contact details) in order to draw a random sample. Binley's (**www.binleys.com/About.asp**), a private UK company, supplies accessible registration lists giving contact details. However, Binley's does not hold named listings of hospital doctors at Foundation 1 and Foundation 2 grades because of the mobility of Foundation doctors. Interviewers in one research project who wanted to speak to such doctors thus had to find another way to gain access. They called general hospital numbers asking to be transferred to a ward. When someone on the ward answered the telephone they asked to be put through to a doctor at Foundation 1 or Foundation 2 grades (GfK NOP Social Research, 2011). However, as Foundation schools/deaneries do have lists of all foundation doctors, it would cause far less inconvenience to ward staff if the interviewers had contacted the deaneries. Do think very carefully about the best way to approach people if you plan to do a small survey.

For observational studies you will need to gain clearance from hospital trusts/ health boards or education authorities before you can negotiate access to key staff with authority to permit you to be 'a fly on the wall'. This is the kind of issue in which local research ethics committees (discussed in Chapter 4) are interested. You might deem that behaviour occurring in public spaces is freely observable but it is not always so easy, as you will discover by doing Activity 5.1.

ACTIVITY 5.1

Identify three 'public spaces' where observation might pose ethical or practical difficulties. Plan how you might negotiate access.

A public library might constitute a public space but access to computers could be blocked to websites deemed 'sensitive'. An undergraduate wanting to use the university library to research a sensitive topic (such as child abuse) should discuss the matter first with library staff to find out about necessary clearances. Similarly, a children's playground in a public park may be patrolled as out of bounds to non-parental adults. Even 'people-watching' from the apparent safety of a kerbside café table may attract hostile attention if someone notes you jotting down notes whenever a person passing by spits or is smoking a cigarette.

If your research involves directly contacting people, once you've made contact you need them to give you informed consent (Chapter 4). They retain the right to withdraw at any stage. Decisions will have to be made about who is told what concerning the reason for the investigator's presence. Suppose you are are studying the effects on the family of car accidents where more than one member of the family has been injured – what happens about child care, the consequences of being off work in order to look after an injured spouse and child at the same time, the non-cook now doing the cooking and cleaning, for instance. While it is easy to identify the families, speaking to the non-injured adult is hard. Do you telephone or see that individual in person? If you contact the non-injured person, he or she might think something is wrong or that you are wanting to discuss something painful and stressful.

It's important for researchers who are participants in the research (as in action research, which is often used in audits or evaluations) to have procedures for them to 'debrief'. This is because stress arises from the tension between participative and observer roles (Lee-Treweek, 2000). Observations of bad practices in health-related/ social care settings are known by all members to be reportable, yet there are instances of poor practice that investigators might want to understand better, particularly if they hold a 'detached observer' stance, where the case is less clear-cut. For instance, you might be interested to observe when fellow students are texting in lectures: do they do so when the lecturer is demonstrating something or only when other students are asking questions? Would you feel uncomfortable if the person next to you asked what you were doing as you tallied (put ticks in columns) texting as 'lecturer time' or 'student time'?

In entering previously unknown settings it's important to be sensitive to the potential impact of local politics and rivalries, so do not ally yourself too closely with one person or group if you can avoid doing so. Remember in your interviews it must be obvious you are neutral. In emotive research projects such as the vouchers for refugees that we discussed in Chapter 4, being aware of the political and personal tensions is important but it is also important to be trusted not to take sides or to become allied to someone very helpful in doing the research, especially if that person is known to hold a particular view.

Now we've explored some of the considerations around access, the following sections will look in more detail at each of the main data collection methods (asking questions, observation and documentary sources).

Asking questions

This section will look at the use of a variety of tools for asking questions: **structured questionnaires**, **interviews** (face-to-face or telephone) and **focus group**s.

Structured questionnaires

Questionnaires are used when you want to collect specific information from a large number of people. They are used in surveys and other quantitative methods but also may be used in other research designs where there is a need for standardised information. Questionnaires are structured to reflect the researcher's interests. They are not expected to elicit anything the person completing the questionnaire might consider to be more relevant. You've probably seen evaluation sheets that didn't ask for your opinion on the things that really mattered to you. Perhaps that impelled you to scribble your thoughts in the margins in the hope someone might take notice of them. Open-ended questions (that do not specify possible answers) can be included in questionnaires, but for reasons that will be explained later, usually they are limited in number if they appear at all.

Questions can be specific because many aspects of the topic are already understood. They are considered to be 'objective' because the same question is asked in the same order for each person completing the questionnaire (this is also true when questionnaires are used in face-to-face conditions, where they are referred to as an **interview schedule**). Where the information needed is more complex or uncertain then other forms of interviews or focus groups are more useful.

ACTIVITY 5.2

Nur is a second-year medical student who is interested in his fellow students' experiences of the preclinical years based in the Science Faculty. He is considering two research questions.

1. Do first- and second-year students feel the clinical days they've attended prepare them adequately for the rotations of six-week-long placements they can expect in their third year?
2. How could the debriefing sessions following the clinical days be best used to build their sense of being prepared?

For which question would you suggest a questionnaire be used?

A questionnaire could be used for the first of the questions to provide quantitative data measuring students' attitudes. Focus groups or interviews would be more helpful in addressing the second question: participants could volunteer ideas and suggestions in the light of their experiences.

You also need to consider how to distribute your questionnaire to get the best response. Questionnaires can be posted but this often results in a low response rate (although enclosing a stamped addressed envelope to return the form can help). The response rate is usually better if they are handed out in a setting where there is time to complete them with a box for the receipt of the completed ones. For example, Nur could hand out his questionnaires to students who arrive early for lectures, or he might invite electronic submissions using an online survey, although they also tend to have low response rates.

Some general principles exist for the production of good questionnaires.

- Keep questions and items short and as simply worded as possible – aim for a maximum completion time of 5–15 minutes to maximise response.

- Ensure that each item and question carries only one idea.

- Use language that is clear, unambiguous and relevant, avoiding negatives and double negatives.

- Use mostly closed questions (where the possible answers are offered to be selected).

- Response formats should be standard (left to right or top to bottom) as can be seen in Figure 5.1.

In the PAST WEEK, did you ever have any of the following symptoms:

8. Increased thirst? .... ☐ No   ☐ Yes   ☐ Don't know

9. Dry mouth?.. ☐ No   ☐ Yes   ☐ Don't know

10. Decreased appetite? .... ☐ No   ☐ Yes   ☐ Don't know

11. Nausea or vomiting? .... ☐ No   ☐ Yes   ☐ Don't know

Figure 5.1 Extract from questionnaire (diabetes).

Source: **patienteducation.stanford.edu/research/diabquest.pdf.**

Closed questions (where a choice of answers is given) can be precoded so processing data is fast. If an online survey tool is used (e.g. Bristol online survey, SurveyMonkey or SurveyGizmo), then the answers can be processed automatically by the survey tool and a report produced for the researcher. Open questions in self-filled questionnaires take time to complete and so are often not answered. If they are answered they take longer to process. They can be interpreted differently by different people with no chance for clarification. Experience with SF-36 (a widely used generic multipurpose short-form health survey with 36 questions about physical and mental health) shows that mixed formats of response choices can confuse respondents and cause missing and inconsistent responses, as many researchers have discovered.

Constructing a questionnaire takes time: getting the wording right, planning the order in which questions are asked and piloting it to identify and correct any problems are all lengthy processes. Unless it is a requirement of the programme you are studying, it is a much better use of your time to find out about and use suitable published questionnaires that have been validated already. It also adds to the knowledge base by making your study comparable with others. Reading research papers in your topic area may give you a lead on their names and ways to access them if your supervisor cannot help. Some questionnaires, but not all, are publicly available. Make contact with researchers in your field of interest to ask for access to unpublished instruments (explain succinctly who you are, what you plan to do and ask if you may use it, or the parts of it that are relevant to your study). It is better to use a tool that has already been used than to start from scratch. Well before data collection you should pilot questionnaires and interview schedules carefully on a group similar to the population to be sampled: this will alert you to any difficulties that people may have in answering the questions, and also give you an idea about logistical matters (such as how long it takes for people to respond, getting access to addresses).

Many questionnaires deal with sensitive subjects, and often the anonymity of a questionnaire is useful in gaining information in these circumstances as it avoids the embarrassment of responding to an interviewer. However, there are ways of dealing with this potential embarrassment even in face-to-face interviews where interviewer and respondent are both present. For instance, the questionnaire could be self-completed at the time and put in an envelope.

Advantages of questionnaires

- Questionnaires are relatively inexpensive and quick to administer.
- Questions are consistently structured with no interviewer variability.
- Large numbers of participants are easier to approach.
- Anonymity can be assured.
- There is flexibility regarding when they are completed.
- The absence of an interviewer means less likelihood of bias through people giving socially acceptable answers.

Disadvantages of questionnaires

- There are limits on how much time participants will give to completing the questionnaire.
- They may not be suitable for people with low reading levels, learning disabilities or those for whom the language of the questionnaire is not their first unless administered by a suitable person (and translation itself may remove the certainty of reliability).
- There is no opportunity to probe further or observe body language that might lead to further questioning.
- As the participant is not seen, there is no certainty the correct person filled in the questionnaire.
- Motivating the participant to complete all the questions is easier to do in person.

Table 5.1 suggests when conducting an interview in person may be preferable to administering a questionnaire, and when logistic considerations (time and cost) may make the questionnaire a better choice.

Table 5.1 Relative merits of holding an interview versus using a questionnaire

Consideration	Interview	Questionnaire
Person needed to collect data	Requires trained interviewers	Requires administration
Is it affordable?	Payment to interviewers, transcription	Postage and printing
Opportunities for personalisation in the situation	Extensive	Limited
Opportunities for probing	Possible	Difficult
Relative magnitude of data reduction	Large (because of coding)	Mainly limited to data entry
The number of respondents who can be reached	Limited	Extensive
Efficiency	Rich data but time-poor	Limited data but time-efficient
Sources of error	Interviewer, instrument, coding, sample	Limited to instrument and sample

Interviews

An interview is much more than a conversation with purpose. There is always a power differential between the interviewer and the interviewee and the situation is never natural. Researchers choosing to interview (whether using structured, semistructured or unstructured formats) must build a relationship with participants so that they feel listened to and respected. The interviewer must be careful not to ask leading questions. Questions that make the respondent uncomfortable should be avoided.

Interviews enable participants to express themselves in their own words and to focus on matters participants identify as important. The interviewer is given an opportunity to follow up responses that seem significant for the investigation although, as this is a dialogue, the participant may choose not to respond. Complex issues can be explored which produce richly detailed ('thick') data. People may talk about matters which they would not write about. When an interview is audio- or video-taped they will generally signal 'this is off the record' or 'I didn't say that'. This must be respected in reporting the findings. Interviews are widely used in qualitative designs such as action research and ethnographic research, but may supplement quantitative studies when unusual or unexpected findings in the data suggest that important variables have not been captured by the questionnaire.

ACTIVITY 5.3

Nur's grandmother has recently recovered from a stroke and has moved into residential care. Now he's interested in exploring the possible impact of such a move. He's thinking about interviewing a resident (not his grandmother), a relative, a care assistant, a care manager and a residential home manager.

What problems do you anticipate this might pose for analysing the data?

Nur's investigation in Activity 5.3 would certainly give a broad range of viewpoints as there are so many different roles, but it would be very difficult to develop an interview schedule with questions that are relevant to all the participants. Analysis could be difficult because responses are likely to be very different, and reporting also would be problematic as it would be difficult to protect anonymity because each of the five people could be identified by their role (Chapter 4). As his practical concern is with how little time he has to conduct the interviews, it would be better to confine his interviews to those residents and care staff willing to talk to him about something both groups will have experience of (such as 'What do new residents find most difficult to adjust to when they first arrive?'). Then he could research the literature with similar respondents to compare their findings with his analysis. This question, because it is asked of both groups in the same way, forms the basis of a structured interview.

Standardised or structured (or semistructured) interviews

Interviews where all respondents are asked preplanned questions in a given order are known as standardised or structured interviews using interview schedules. These are generally used for quantitative research, but may also have a part to play in other designs where it is useful to collect data systematically for later comparison (though often this is also fulfilled by semistructured interviews, where more leeway is given to probe further with follow-up questions). An example of questions in a structured interview showing the instructions to the interviewer follows.

---

1 (a). Do you use the *library itself*, on average: (read out the options and tick one)

    ❑ Less than once a month
    ❑ Once a month
    ❑ Once every two weeks
    ❑ Once a week
    ❑ Two or three times a week
    ❑ Daily

1 (b). Do you ever use the *library services via the internet* on a computer that is in *another location* to the library, e.g. at home, at work, at college?

    ❑ Yes
    ❑ No

Many of the issues regarding questions on a questionnaire also apply to interview schedules. Yet because they are administered by a trained interviewer, interview schedules can be much more complex. Large-scale surveys employ teams of researchers to carry out interviews. To ensure **reliability** (replicability), interview schedules contain full instructions for the interviewer in order to maximise consistency in how different interviewers conduct the interview. Interviewers are also usually trained together for the same reasons.

Unstructured interviews

An unstructured interview contains many open-ended questions, which are not asked in a structured, precise manner. Different researchers interpret questions and often offer different explanations when respondents ask for clarification. Different respondents may be asked different questions and the interviewer is free to probe further in order to gain more insights. Nur might find he wants to ask some follow-up questions so as to be certain he has understood what he is being told. 'When you say "the meals", what do you mean exactly – is it the food itself or the times they are served or what?'

Unstructured interviews may involve just a single question or be a list of topics that need to be covered. This tool is used by researchers adopting a phenomeno-logical approach (a psychological paradigm researching how members of a particular group perceive their experiences; see Chapter 1, Figure 1.5). They usually draw on interviews or on personal written accounts for data. In the hands of an experienced researcher who has identified a **key informant** (a person who is very knowledgeable about a situation) it could be very productive to ask *What sensory feedback do you get from your prosthesis? How does your experience of using your prosthesis now differ to when you first began using one? Have you/do you experience a phantom limb? Can you tell me about these experiences?* (Murray, 2004, p965). Since the phenomenologist is interested in how the other person's world is experienced, the questions that elicit this information can't be foretold. So a structured interview is inappropriate.

For novices, this tool is risky. You can easily accumulate a series of transcripts (or field notes) of diverse individual interviews that prove difficult to analyse. However, as a starting point for undertaking an audit or a health service evaluation this could be an excellent beginning. Finding a key informant who knows the issues, the people to contact and how to go about it solves many logistical problems.

Incidentally, just as quantitative researchers take into account how they will analyse their data when finalising their study design, so too do qualitative researchers have to consider how detailed the transcripts of the interviews should be. For ethnographers (who study people in their social setting in order to describe their customs, beliefs and behaviour), simply typing out the words of an interview will be sufficient transcription along with their field notes. However, for conversation analysis and some other forms of discourse analysis where recordings of human interaction are not just listened to or looked at but are empirically examined for how meaning is constructed, textual transcription includes signs that conventionally signal timings, length of pauses, overlap of speech and rise and fall of intonation. It takes about five to six times as long as a recording lasts simply to type it out; it can take very much longer to add in the detail of the sounds as they are uttered. If accompanied by gestures recorded on video, it takes much longer still.

An example of a section of transcribed recording follows in the box below.

Example of transcription AD Grandson Black Eye (see Table 5.2)

```
 1. CPO:      Is that o[↑ka:y.]
 2. Caller:        [ Fine.] =yes.
 3.           [°that's fine.°]
 4. CPO:      [↓Brilliant  ] okay,
 5. Caller:  °.Hh° (0.2) u:m (0.1) >I'm sorry
 6.          I'm a little bit< emo:~tional
 7.          to↑d[ay~ .hih]
 8. CPO:         [Tch Oh::] go:sh I'm so:rry,
 9. Caller:  ~I've got a little four year old grandson,~
10.          [huh]
11. CPO:     [Yea]h:,
12.          (0.3)
13. Caller:  ~My son w(h)as s(h)ixtee:n~ (0.5) er fif↓teen when
14.          he was bor:n.
15.          (0.3)
```

www-staff.lboro.ac.uk/~ssjap/transcription/transcription.htm

Table 5.2 Examples of common transcription conventions originally developed by Gail Jefferson

[	A single left bracket indicates the point of overlap onset
]	A single right bracket indicates the point at which an utterance or utterance part terminates vis-à-vis another
=	Equal signs, one at the end of one line and one at the beginning of a next, indicate no 'gap' between the two lines. This is often called latching
(0.0)	Numbers in parentheses indicate elapsed time in silence by tenth of seconds, so (7.1) is a pause of 7 seconds and one-tenth of a second
word	Underscoring indicates some form of stress, via pitch and/or amplitude; an alternative method is to print the stressed part in italics

Source: ten Have (2007) **www.paultenhave.nl/Transcription-DCA-2.htm**

If you read the sample transcript following Jefferson's conventions you will reproduce what was heard by the person who transcribed the extract from a recording. Jefferson was developing a line of research already started by a colleague, Harvey Sacks, who was tragically killed in a car crash. Much of what we know about the interviewing process comes from the close attention it has received from sociological research which draws extensively on this data collection method, as the case study below demonstrates.

Case study: Influences on data collection – quotes from Harvey Sacks' lectures

Harvey Sacks (1935–75) was a famous American sociologist who became interested in the structure of conversation in the 1960s while working at a (tape-recorded) suicide counselling hotline.

> *When I started to do research in sociology I figured that sociology could not be an actual science unless it was able to handle the details of actual events, handle them formally, and in the first instance be informative about them in the direct ways in which primitive sciences tend to be informative – that is, that anyone else can go and see whether what was said is so. And that is a tremendous control on seeing whether one is learning anything.*
>
> *I started to work with tape-recorded conversations. Such materials had a single virtue, that I could replay them. I could transcribe them somewhat and study them extendedly – however long it might take. The tape-recorded materials constituted a 'good enough' record of what happened. Other things, to be sure, happened, but at least what was on the tape had happened. It was not from any large interest in language or from some theoretical formulation of what should be studied that I started with tape-recorded conversations, but simply because I could get my hands on it and I could study it again and again, and also, consequentially, because others could look at what I had studied and make of it what they could, if, for example, they wanted to be able to disagree with me.*
>
> (Sacks, 1984, p26, from a lecture given in the autumn of 1967)

This extract makes it clear that Sacks worked within a positivist paradigm. By tape-recording interviews Sacks opened the way for very sophisticated and close analysis of how people construct meaning through talk (a form of qualitative research known as conversation analysis). In learning 'how to break bad news' you are drawing on the careful observation of how doctors prepare their patient (the hesitation and the tone for instance), that originates from this approach to knowledge.

Considerations for face-to-face and telephone interviews

Before you conduct an interview, whether it is structured, semistructured or unstructured, there are some things you should consider. Notice that with telephone interviews you depend on voice (tone, enthusiasm, pace and pitch) and there are no overt body language cues. They are well suited to structured, directed questioning using quantitative methods. On the other hand, face-to-face interviews allow you to build the rapport that is needed in qualitative research.

Preparation for any type of interview is important. We have listed some of the key considerations below.

1. At recruitment, brief your interviewees.
   In getting their consent for participation you should provide them with information about the investigation.

   - Make sure they understand why you want to interview them and what you will use their information or views for.

   - Assure them of confidentiality.

   - Tell them how long the interview should take.

   - Agree a time and place for the interview that are mutually convenient. Ensure the location is comfortable or familiar to the interviewee and that there is privacy.

   - Ensure the interviewee knows who you are and how to contact you.

2. Just before the interview.

   - Ensure you have all the equipment you need (take spare tapes and batteries if you are going to record the interview and check everything is working).

   - Check again that your questions cover all the information you need.

   - Check the environment is suitable for the interview.

   - Make sure you know where you're going and allow time for getting lost if it's new to you.

3. When the interview starts:

   - Break the ice with a little friendly chat if you don't know them already, to help make them comfortable and establish a rapport. Remind them of who you are and the purpose of the investigation. Make it clear they do not have to answer any questions if they don't want to and how confidentiality and anonymity will be assured.

   - If it is a face-to-face interview, be aware of your body language and notice theirs. Make sure you are attentive and interested so as to build rapport. If they are looking uncomfortable, look at them in a friendly understanding way and reassure them that their answers are valid and confidential.

   - Speak clearly and let the respondent know you're listening. Use words and sounds to show this (Uh, mmm, OK, for instance – but avoid approving words like 'definitely' that might influence later responses). This is especially important for telephone interviews.

   - Follow up to clarify points if necessary but remember to stick to the agreed time – they may have a child to collect from school or another appointment.

Often, however, people will be prepared to spend longer, or be willing to be contacted again (if you ask).

- Thank participants for their time and make notes of key points and thoughts that occur to you. Store data securely.

Although telephone interviews have been used successfully in qualitative investigation, particularly where people are hard to reach (Dadich and Muir, 2009; Tausig and Freeman, 1988), they have been displaced by the use of e-mail interviews in many circumstances (Dommeyer and Moriarty, 2000; Meho, 2006). Table 5.3 outlines the advantages and disadvantages of using e-mail for interviews.

Table 5.3 Advantages/disadvantages of e-mail interviewing

	Advantages	*Disadvantages*
Interviewers and participants	Allows access to: • Those difficult or impossible to reach or interview face to face or via telephone • Those individuals who cannot express themselves as well in talking as they do in writing • Those who prefer online interaction over face-to-face or telephone conversation	Limited to individuals with access to the internet Requires skills in online communication from both interviewer and interviewees Requires expertise in technology from both interviewer and interviewees
Cost	Costs of calling, travelling, transcribing, recruiting large/geographically dispersed samples substantially reduced	Time costs are displaced to participants
Time	Eliminates time required for transcribing, scheduling appointments Allows interviewing more than one participant at a time	May take several days or weeks before an interview is complete
Recruitment	Done via e-mail, listservs, message boards, discussion groups, and/or web pages	Invitations for participation may be deleted before they are read
Participation	Done by e-mail	High undeliverable rates (e.g. due to inactive e-mail addresses)
Medium effects	Allows participants to take part in the interviews in a familiar environment (e.g. home or office); to take their time in answering questions; to express their opinions and feelings more honestly (because of sense of anonymity) Encourages self-disclosure Eliminates interruption that takes place in face-to-face/telephone interviews	Empowers participants, essentially allowing them to be in control of the flow of the interview Does not allow direct probing Requires that questions be more self-explanatory than those posed face to face or by telephone, to avoid miscommunication and misinterpretation

	Eliminates transcription errors	Loses visual and non-verbal cues due to
	Eliminates interviewer/interviewee	inability to read facial expressions or
	effect resulting from visual and non-	body languages or hear the voice tones
	verbal cues or status difference between	of each other
	the two (e.g. race, gender, age, voice	May narrow participants'
	tones, dress, gestures, disabilities)	interpretations and, thereby, constrain
	Cues and emotions can be conveyed	their responses
	through use of certain symbols or text	Requires meticulous attention to detail
		Participants may lose focus
Data quality	Allows participants to construct their	One-dimensional (based on text only)
	own experiences with their own dialogue	Indepth information is not always easily
	and interaction with the researcher	obtainable
	Facilitates a closer connection with	
	interviewee's personal feelings, beliefs,	
	and values	
	Data are more focused on the interview	
	questions asked	
	Responses are more thought out before	
	they are sent	

Source: Meho (2006, p1292). Reproduced with permission.

Group interviews

Focus groups are group interviews, widely used in evaluation research. The tool is favoured by action researchers but it is also used in mixed-methods studies (Chapters 1 and 4).

Similar challenges occur as in face-to-face interviews. The role of the facilitator (who may or may not be the researcher) is vital. The facilitator initially tries to promote a relaxed atmosphere so people feel comfortable talking in the group. Facilitators might, for example, hand out refreshments as participants arrive. Generally a group size of four to seven people works well.

A general unthreatening question is asked first and there will be a list of topic areas (and prompts) for the facilitator to use if they are not addressed spontaneously by participants. Participants' responses evoke sharing of experiences and attitudes or may challenge what is said. This provides rich data. However, it's important to remember the context of the data production. Utterances cannot be presented as the essential 'views' of the participants. Group members may say things simply because they are part of the group. For example, perhaps they are feeling peer pressure and wish to be seen to be going along with what others are saying. Also, sometimes individual members can dominate and influence others in groups. In other words, group dynamics will play a part and need to be taken into account. To bring up a range of different perceptions, focus groups need to have a mix of people who have not met before. An example of how a focus group can be used to explore sensitive health topics follows in 'What's the evidence?'

What's the evidence?

Focus groups were used in a study to explore issues of resilience and positive out-comes among a group of 12 individuals with a range of visible differences (psoriasis, port wine stain, scarring, amputations, burn injuries, impact of thyroid eye disease, mastectomy, alopecia and altered appearance of their hands or nose). The following extract shows how a focus group worked in practice.

Participants in the focus group interviews talked openly both to the interviewer and to each other about their experiences. They were responding to points that others had made and the interaction was clearly beneficial in terms of the amount of data generated. Small groups allowed participants to build a good rapport with others and gave them confidence to ask each other personal questions, which they may not have felt comfortable doing in a larger group. The current study supports Frith's (2000) assertion that focus groups are ideal for gaining knowledge on issues that are under-researched, including sensitive topics. Additionally, this study supports Frith's point that researchers are able to get an awareness of the strength with which particular views are held and to understand the ways in which participants defend and rationalize these views. Although one could argue that the study included a motivated sample, as the participants had previously taken part in appearance-related research, none of the participants in the group interviews had attended one before, and they gave a large amount of positive feedback to the researcher, for example by expressing that it had been 'useful for them', they were 'happy to help', and 'glad they had come'. This suggests that focus groups are not only beneficial in terms of data collection but that they can also be a valuable experience for those who take part.

(Egan et al., 2011, p746)

Another type of group interview, called the **nominal group** technique, is oriented to establishing consensus and is favoured for doing clinical improvement. It uses a highly structured meeting with key informants to gather information about a given issue. Key informants discuss and then usually rate and re-rate a series of items or questions. Provided the interview is conducted sensitively it is usually well accepted. Ideally, these types of interviews should be carried out by a person with local knowledge who works in the facility or in a similar one. Whilst this is not a tool that can precisely measure the extent of a problem, it is useful for finding out what people subjectively feel is a problem that needs to be addressed. So they are useful for setting common shared priorities for things like patient safety initiatives (World Health Organization, 2010, p7).

Learning how to ask patients questions that will elicit answers that are helpful to you in making a diagnosis, as well as managing the interaction to be both efficient and respectful, are skills you develop as a medical student. How is what you have read in this section 'Asking Questions' covering different approaches to interviewing, any different from what you are expected to do as a medical student taking a case history? We now move on to discuss another way of collecting data, namely observation.

Observation

Eyewitness accounts are valued for knowing 'what is going on here'. Observation usually means both watching and listening, although it may entail just one of these. Observation as a tool for generating data is based on the following characteristics.

- Events, actions and meanings are viewed from the standpoint of the people being studied (the **emic perspective**).

- Events and actions must be placed in their social and historical setting to understand them.

- Attention should be paid to detail.

- The observer tries not to infer meanings prematurely, and attempts to recognise that activities are not discrete events but are part of a bigger process.

Observation takes place in laboratory and clinical settings as well as within organisations and communities. Records may take the form of completed checklists or data sheets, laboratory notebooks, diaries and field notes, photographs, audio or video tapes and their transcriptions. It's important to remember that records are constructed – elements have been selected and presented in a way that makes sense to the researcher. Participant observation differs from structured observation in that, in order to develop understanding of the purpose and meaning of what is observed, the participant observer becomes partially socialised to the group being studied.

Participant observation

Living among those being researched so as to share activities with a group's members is referred to as fieldwork. In ethnography researchers do fieldwork where they engage in varying degrees of participation and observation (often in combination with formal interviews and reading documents).

Negotiating access to the research 'field' can prove problematic as often there are gatekeepers to satisfy. Studies attempting to explore service users' views and experiences of their treatment, for example, could be derailed by a gatekeeper manager who is defensively reluctant to have user 'complaints' researched by a stranger – a factor that is worth bearing in mind when doing clinical audit or health service evaluation (Chapters 9 and 10).

Observations that are naturalistic require your presence to be unregarded by others. How you dress and behave therefore becomes important. Nowadays the use of videos to record details of interactions, such as those between healthcare providers and users, extends the possibilities for analysis but also creates new ethical issues regarding its future use. While consent will have been sought and granted for such recordings to take place, having the camera in place before recording helps participants get used to its presence. It also helps if you mask any light that shows when the camera is 'live' (Haw and Hadfield, 2011). The aim is to encourage people to act naturally, which they do once they forget the interaction is being recorded, so it is important that participants are comfortable with the idea that the record will continue to exist to be reviewed in the future, and they have consented to the purposes for which it will be used. Issues of confidentiality and anonymity become harder to sustain when an audience who may have knowledge of the participants widens (because they are all within a medical community that could access the video). Advice can be found on the General Medical Council (GMC) website: **www.gmc-uk.org/guidance/ethical_guidance/ making_audiovisual.asp**. In most circumstances, and where necessary, covert recordings should only be carried out by the police.

Another challenge for those doing fieldwork relates to the degree of researcher participation. This challenge comes to the fore in 'covert' field studies where researchers run the risk of participating rather than simply observing. A covert study might be needed to find out about people's behaviour, as with observing doctors' hand-washing behaviour (Haessler *et al.*, 2012). Like 'secret shoppers' who monitor on behalf of chain stores the service they receive at a particular outlet (Krevor *et al.*, 2011), 'clients' were sent into pharmacies in Accra, Ghana to find out if pharmacists were following the Ministry of Health's guidelines about the advice they were supposed to give about different forms of contraception. The use of 'simulated patients' is widely used for monitoring pharmacy practice (Watson *et al.*, 2006).

Activity 5.4 asks you to think how a participant observer might be used to improve the quality of care.

ACTIVITY 5.4

As a medical student you are well placed as a participant to observe the professional behaviour of fellow students towards patients and others.

How could you use this to improve healthcare delivery?

This activity could identify poor practice. If it did, the next step would be to find out how to improve matters. In a qualitative study relevant for this step, Garner *et al.* (2010) investigated medical school student views on peer assessment of professional behaviour by conducting focus groups in two English medical schools that used such peer assessment. Such assessments were based on participant observation. It is interesting to note, however, that giving feedback electronically was preferred by some because it could be done anonymously. It *can give a true picture, but keep to a limit 'cause it's as if I want to be harsh but it's not . . . it's more about giving someone proper constructive feedback* (Garner *et al.*, 2010, p34). Others suggested it was better given face to face because then it was possible to explain and discuss behaviour more fully.

Structured observation

Structured observation is a systematic method of data collection, where there is considerable precoding and the observation takes the form of recording when, how often or for how long the precoded behaviours occur. As with structured questionnaires, this tool yields quantitative results. It's been used widely in the study of hygiene behaviour, and for water contact behaviour in relation to schistosomiasis transmission (Cheesmond and Fenwick, 1981). When people are questioned about the disposal of infants' faeces, questionnaire data were found to be less valid than data obtained by direct observation. Questionnaires overreport socially acceptable behaviour (Curtis *et al.*, 1993).

To construct this tool the range of possible behaviours is defined during a preliminary study. A precoded data collection form is produced, and observers are trained to use these forms. Data collection is time-consuming, so sites and times for observation are usually sampled. Figure 5.2 shows an extract of an observation form for a medical student's interaction with a child and family.

Behavior	Child	Family
Uses names of family members and children		
Incorporates social talk in the beginning of the visit		
Shows interest and attention		
Demonstrates empathy		
Appears patient and unhurried		

Figure 5.2 Extract from *Observation Form Effective Behaviors in Patient- or Family-Centered Communication.* **www.pediatricsinpractice.org/pdfs/Communication/Communication_handout 3-3-r.pdf**

The person completing this form will have been trained to recognise each of the items to ensure reliability (as happened with training interviewers using interview schedules).

An example of an observation tool for hand-washing and the accompanying instructions for how to use it can be found at **www.idrn.org/nosec/Hand% 20hygiene%20observation%20tool1.pdf** and **www.idrn.org/nosec/ IDRN%20HHO%20training.pdf**

Laboratory notebooks are an example of structured observations that have to be meticulously maintained. Everyone should keep detailed records of the experiments conducted each day.

The precise way in which to document scientific research varies from field to field and from institution to institution, but some general rules apply, such as the following:

- *Use a permanently bound book, with consecutive signed and dated entries. When appropriate, witness entries as well.*

- *For computer-kept logs, you can use a loose-leaf notebook, but pages must be consecutively numbered (using a sequential page-number stamp), dated, and signed. Record entries chronologically. Each entry should stand on its own to permit others to replicate the work.*

- *Organise material with sections and headings.*

- *Identify and describe reagents and specimens used.*

- *Identify sources of those materials (e.g., reagent manufacturer, lot number, purity, expiration date).*

- *Enter instrument serial numbers and calibration dates.*

- *Use proper nouns for items.*

- *Write all entries in the first person, and be specific about who did the work.*

- *Explain nonstandard abbreviations.*

- *Use ink and never obliterate original writing; never remove pages or portions of a page.*

- *If a page is left blank or a space within a page is left blank, draw a line through it.*

- *Permanently affix with glue any attachments (such as graphs or computer print-outs) to the pages of the notebook; date and sign both the notebook page and the attachment.*

- *Outline new experiments, including their objectives and rationale.*

- *Include periodic factual, not speculative, summaries of status and findings.*

- *Enter ideas and observations into your notebook immediately. Summarise discussions from lab meetings and ideas or suggestions made by others, citing the persons by name.*

(Howard Hughes Medical Institute and Burroughs Wellcome Fund,
2006, p145)

Documentary sources

As well as asking questions and observing behaviour (primary data), data can also be collected from a variety of documentary sources. These sources of data include public records (government documents, minutes of meeting, as shown in Table 5.4), private documents (medical histories, diaries) as well as transcripts from interviews or observational data. Routinely collected data such as patient records and hospital activity analysis are used with clinical audits and health service evaluation. Note that archives may not be complete (fire, flood or moving premises: all can lose material).

Table 5.4 Sources of secondary data

Type of data required	UK sources
Demographic and lifestyle data	Census, General Household Survey, social trends, annual reports
Mortality data	ONS mortality statistics
Morbidity data	GP morbidity statistics, communicable disease surveillance, hospital inpatient inquiry, hospital activity analysis, cancer registration
Health services data	Immunisation data, screening levels, district and annual reports, confidential inquiry reports
Specific databases	ONS survey of disability, ONS longitudinal study, abortion data, congenital abnormalities
Other	Work and pensions statistics, commissions of inquiry

Source: Office for National Statistics (ONS): **www.ons.gov.uk/ons/index.html**.

A major source of healthcare information is hospital activity analysis. Activity analysis breaks down what goes on in hospitals into discrete activities independently of how they are organised (admissions, appointments, diagnoses and discharges, for instance). Data for this analysis are anonymised, coded and forwarded by a hospital's patient administration system (PAS) to a central dataset Secondary Uses Service (SUS) that provides information to Hospital Episode Statistics (HES) (**www. hesonline.nhs.uk/Ease/servlet/ContentServer?siteID=1937**). Additional data may be available for certain specialties, from pathology or radiology systems, for instance.

Coding clinical data

Clinical coding is the process whereby information written in the patient notes is translated into coded data and entered onto hospital information systems. Coding usually occurs after the patient has been discharged from hospital, and must be completed to strict deadlines in order for hospitals to receive payment for their activity.

Clinical coding staff are entirely dependent on clear, accurate information about all diagnoses and procedures in order to produce a true picture of hospital activity. The coded data are vitally important, and are used for:

- *Monitoring the provision of health services across the UK*
- *Research and the monitoring of health trends and variations*
- *NHS financial planning and Payment by Results*
- *Local and national clinical audit and case-mix analysis*
- *Clinical governance.*

(www.ic.nhs.uk/webfiles/Clinical/Hospital_Activity_Data_ A_Guide_for_Clinicians_England.pdf)

PAS data are collected primarily to support corporate and administrative processes, as you can see by their content. Information is fed back to consultants (and through them to their teams) that can inform their practice but there may be discrepancies between the analysis and actual practice for a variety of reasons. For instance, where practice is largely outpatient-based few practical clinical procedures might be recorded.

In appraising documentary sources, issues of authorship (who wrote it?) and the expected audience are important matters to think about (as discussed in Chapter 8). These can limit the richness and verisimilitude of the data (how like the 'real thing' it is). For instance, the minutes of a meeting written by an administrator will not look much like the field notes of the short-hand-proficient investigator who was allowed to be present at the meeting. The administrator's notes will record decisions taken; the investigator's will also note body language and the process of decision-making, for example.

Many rich sources of documentary data arise from blogs and discussion groups on the internet. All those involved in healthcare (staff, carers and patients) can bene-fit from the use of 'reflective digital storytelling' as an educational methodology. The Pilgrim Projects' 'Patient Voices' provides a rich archive of such materials, as you will see in Activity 5.5. Note, however, that the ease with which you can access such data does not absolve you from your professional obligation to respect ethics and patient confidentiality and to use your observations professionally.

ACTIVITY 5.5

Visit the Patient Voices website **www.patientvoices.org.uk/stories.htm** and click on the link to 'Reconnecting with life: stories of life after stroke'.

How might Nur use this to understand better the experiences of his grandmother and other residents in her new accommodation?

This is rich documentary evidence, though in digital form. *The patients, carers and professionals who contributed their stories to the Patient Voices programme have consented to their use as an educational and learning resource as part of the international drive to improve the quality and responsiveness of services for patients and carers.* However, unless such resources are used for that purpose a valuable aim will fail to be realised.

Data quality

Asking questions, observing and documentary sources are all forms of data collec-tion. Regardless of how data were collected, we need to trust the results of research, which is why we evaluate it against criteria that are important to the paradigm we favour. When evaluating their own work, qualitative researchers use different crite-ria from those used by quantitative researchers. Quantitative researchers use criteria such as reliability, validity and generalisability. Instead, qualitative researchers use criteria more responsive to their specific research paradigm, such as 'ethical integ-rity', 'rigour', 'authenticity', 'relevance', 'coherence' and 'artistry', as well as validity (Finlay, 2006).

Quantitative measures of data quality

Reliability is about the extent to which repeated measurements using the same research technique under the same conditions produce the same results. Reliability is tested by repetition, so that the most reliable results are those that can be repeated on several occasions with a similar but different sample.

Validity means how far a study properly measures what it is meant to. For example, to test the hypothesis that a ban on smoking in public places will reduce lung cancer rates, a direct relationship between the two needs to be established for research to be valid.

Generalisability exists when the results of the research can be applied more generally and more widely than the research study itself.

Qualitative measures of data quality

All research methods are concerned about validity. In qualitative research it's important to discriminate between:

- the description of the setting and the processes observed and asked about;

and

- the views and the analysis of the researcher (Popay *et al.*, 1998).

Problems of validity arise when tools for data collection do not accurately represent actual behaviour (Curtis *et al.*, 1993). Researching socially sensitive behaviour such as sexual activity or alcohol consumption suffers from these problems. What actually happens is more likely to be picked up by some ways of collecting data than others. In a study of sexual habits in the Gambia, Pickering *et al.* (1992) concluded that **key informant** interviews produced more valid data than did structured interviews with prostitutes. The term 'key informant' refers to individuals who can provide detailed information and opinion based on their knowledge of a particular issue (such as the clients of prostitutes).

One way to test the validity of data is to triangulate it. **Triangulation** involves using more than one method to produce different forms of data (or the same method to gather data from different sources). The data can be compared, and similar findings from different methods may support the validity and comprehensiveness of the research findings. Triangulation permits assessment of how far accounts overlap. In addition comparing different sources about the same issue under investigation helps to reveal different facets of the phenomenon.

'Ethical integrity', 'rigour', 'authenticity', 'relevance', 'coherence' and 'artistry' all relate to how well the research describes and explains the lived experiences of those people who are being studied.

Storing your data

You have now collected your data. The data should be locked away securely (and anonymised with the key password protected and kept elsewhere). Remember the GMC's stance on patient details found outside hospital: you must use encrypted flash drives. All data should be anonymised, stored securely, with access only to yourself and your supervisor. Remember, you'll have to organise the data well so that when you come to analyse the results you can find what you are looking for easily and go back and add missing data that you could not find the first time. Generally research data should be stored securely for as long as the data may be needed – for publicly funded research this is at least ten years.

Chapter summary

This chapter described:

- how to gain access to people and places;

- that the appropriateness of the tool (method or instrument) depends on your purpose and study design;

- that the tools for finding out are asking questions, observation and documentary sources;

- that data quality criteria differ for quantitative and qualitative investigations;

- that data should be anonymised and stored securely;

- that in order to collect reliable data you have to gain the trust of the people from whom you are collecting data. You need to be absolutely clear about what you want to know, why this information is important and how you plan to analyse the data.

GOING FURTHER

Economic and Social Data Service (ESDS): **www.esds.ac.uk/about/about.asp**
   This portal of entry to online databases and learning guides to key economic and social data, both quantitative and qualitative, spans many disciplines and themes.

ESDS Qualidata: **www.esds.ac.uk/qualidata/support/teachingpacks.asp**
   This gives access to learning materials for data collection. Each data collection method comes with real-life examples of data from an ESDS Qualidata study. The

third resource is based on secondary analysis of qualitative data and showcases Peter Townsend's Last Refuge *study to demonstrate how data can be reused.*

Hamilton, RJ and Bowers, BJ (2006) Internet recruitment and e-mail interviews in qualitative studies. *Qualitative Health Research,* 16 (6): 821–835.
This is a useful and detailed account of key issues. It is worthwhile scanning the table of contents of more recent copies of this journal to see what topics are attracting interest.

Howard Hughes Medical Institute and Burroughs Wellcome Fund (2006) *Making the Right Moves: A practical guide to scientific management for postdocs and new faculty,* 2nd edition. **www.hhmi.org/labmanagement.**
Proper recording of laboratory activities and managing the volumes of data produced by a laboratory are becoming increasingly important. Chapter 8 covers some of the basics: the importance of day-to-day record-keeping and good practice for laboratory notebooks, what to consider when developing a system to track and store information, and finding the right data management system for you.

Pilgrim Projects 'Patient Voices' **www.patientvoices.org.uk/stories.htm**
Bookmark this site as a source of relevant case materials for patient-centred care and ideas for your own research studies/teaching in the future.

chapter 6

Data Processing and Analysis
Ann K. Allen with Blanche Lumb and Michael Hollifield

Achieving your medical degree

This chapter will help you to begin to meet the following requirements of *Tomorrow's Doctors* (General Medical Council, 2009).

Outcomes 1 – The doctor as a scholar and a scientist

10. Apply social science principles, method and knowledge to medical practice.

    (c) Apply theoretical frameworks of sociology to explain the varied responses of individuals, groups and societies to disease.

12. Apply scientific method and approaches to medical research.

The chapter will also enable you to meet the UK Foundation Curriculum (Academy of Medical Royal Colleges, 2012) requirements for engaging in and understanding research, audit and evaluation.

Chapter overview

This chapter will help you to organise and analyse all your data to achieve your research aims. After reading this chapter you will be able to:

- prepare data for analysis;
- construct a coding frame;
- explain basic principles of classification and measurement;
- produce tables and other means to summarise data and present data clearly and appropriately;
- plan your analysis and make an accurate and meaningful interpretation of study findings.

Introduction

You probably thought that planning your investigation was a hurdle until you started to collect your data. Then, issues of access and maintaining momentum in the face of unanticipated difficulties made planning seem the easy stage. And now comes the daunting moment of confronting a mass of figures and results from lab books or data sheets, dog-eared questionnaires, transcripts or field notes (or their electronic equivalent). Somehow they need to be sorted and ordered and summarised in a way that makes sense (to you and others) and addresses the reason why you started in the first place. You perhaps wanted to describe what is happening (as with a descriptive survey), to evaluate what is happening (as with health service evaluation, clinical audit or quality improvement) or to explain your observations either by testing a hypothesis from quantitative data using appropriate statistics, or by generating grounded theory out of qualitative data.

Whatever your purpose, data analysis involves a mixture of common sense, technical expertise and sheer curiosity. As is the case with the research design and methods, the analysis and interpretation of the study should relate to the study's objectives and research questions. In qualitative studies, analysis proceeds alongside data collection. With quantitative investigations, analysis follows data collection (though, as you have seen in Chapter 1, you anticipated the analytic stage when designing your study and you'll be keeping an eye on your results as they accumulate). This will have enabled you to pre-code many of the answers to questions in your questionnaire, but there may have been some open-ended questions that will need to be coded (an analytical process in which data are categorised to facilitate analysis). Clearly the details will differ but, regardless of the methodology you adopted, there are common processes associated with data analysis and interpretation that this chapter will address. Before you can start analysing, though, there's usually a considerable amount of preparatory work to be done.

Preparing data for analysis

Periodic checks of the raw data in laboratory notebooks mean you can uncover and correct carelessness before it becomes a big problem. It's important where errors have occurred that you do not delete or erase the mistake. Correct the data at the point in the log when the error was discovered and refer to the original page – entries should be dated and signed.

We've all spent considerable time designing the perfect study and found that our data are hopelessly flawed – you don't have enough fully completed questionnaires, the questions were misinterpreted, you didn't collect data from the people you intended to and now all your questionnaire responses have a strong bias, your interview transcripts are too difficult to decipher and garbled. If your questions did not provide the data you need to meet your study objectives, you'll have to start again. If your questions were ambiguous, you'll have to discard them. If you did not have an adequate number of responses, you'll have to get more (by combining categories rather than soliciting more respondents). The earlier you recognise any flaws in your study design and data collection, the more time you will save during analysis.

Preparing your data involves a number of tasks best approached systematically (and ideally at the time they are actually collected, not later).

1. Check and order the collected data.

2. Construct a **coding frame** – finding a way to code your data.

3. Code (including double-checking) and construct a **data matrix**.

Check and order the data

You should number and check questionnaires and transcripts for legibility and completeness. The number can incorporate digits giving relevant information about the respondent, such as '01' to signal a first-year medical student. You should also ensure records are anonymised and locked away securely – all computer files should be secured by a password.

You should then check the answers to questionnaires: any blanks might mean they were unasked, unanswerable or inapplicable. If you are checking within hours of an interview a quick telephone call to the interviewer may resolve the issue. Unlike the coding process, checking must be done one questionnaire/interview at a time so the checker has the best possible picture of the respondent. Inconsistencies between answers to different factual questions may highlight a problem. A 20-year-old student is unlikely to have a pension. It's possible other answers may resolve whether the answer to a question about age or income source is correct; for instance, if there were other questions asking about marital status and hobbies, the responses 'widowed' and 'bowls' might suggest 'pension' was right as the source of income, so you would check if the poorly written 20 might be 70. If answers to other questions do not help in this way then the answers to both questions will be 'unknown'.

Where there are missing data it's important to code this with a number that could not also be a true figure (so the computer will not read it as anything other than missing data). If your respondents are all medical students, then 99 is probably a good number – no one is likely to be that old.

When a respondent answers an 'other, please specify' question by selecting 'other' and then writes in an answer that was one of the listed response options, you need to correct this. For instance, a demographic question asking for the respondent's role within the organisation may offer precoded responses like 'administrator, teacher, student or other (please specify)'. If on the questionnaire 'other' is ticked but 'senior lecturer' given, then you would want to clean the response by switching the 'other' choice to the one for 'teacher'. If you didn't do this then the 'other' response will be overstated and the correct response will be understated.

You should record how often a question poses a problem. The frequency might suggest that the question was misunderstood either by the respondent or by the interviewer. If data collection is still in progress then interviewers can be contacted and coached. This may make it difficult to compare answers, however, and if data collection has ceased then treat answers to that particular question cautiously. This is why it is so important to pilot questionnaires and interview schedules carefully on a group similar to the population to be sampled well before data collection.

Electronic surveys throw up the issue of duplicate responses. To find duplicate responses, carefully examine the answers to any open-ended questions. When two open-ended questions have exactly the same answer, a duplicate response is likely to exist. Make sure the response is indeed a duplicate by comparing the answers to all the other questions, and then delete one of the responses if a match is found.

An important part of what you do in this process is to assess the potential for bias (arising because of non-response, refusal and loss, and differences between comparison groups if you have them in your study). Bias was discussed in Chapter 3.

Construct a coding frame

Coding is an analytical process in which data are categorised to aid analysis. One code should apply to only one category and categories should be comprehensive. Codes are entered into a database for analysis (or more low-tech means, such as coloured pens or annotations, can be used for small amounts of data). The aim is to create variables from data, with an eye towards their analysis.

The set of rules for classifying either what was written in transcripts of interviews or questionnaire responses is known as the coding frame. This is a systematic way of classifying data that must be adhered to if useful information is to be generated. The rules for classifying answers or other forms of data are determined by the purpose of the investigation. For instance, all doctors when completing a death certificate refer to the World Health Organization's *International Classification of Diseases* (1994). Examples of other types of coding frame are given in Table 6.1. The numbers (representing a defined category) are entered in the database for analysis. For large amounts of data this makes retrieval quicker and more reliable than dots made on paper records by coloured pens to be tallied up by hand. Qualitative data software such as NVivo or ATLAS.ti tags text so that it can be retrieved and re-examined in context.

Table 6.1 Extracts from two coding frames

Extract from a coding frame relating to answers on a questionnaire about religion (the number is the code entered in the database)

10 Religious Society of Friends/Quaker
11 Other Protestant
   (including: Lutheran Council of Britain; Evangelical Lutheran Churches; Churches of Christ; Churches of Overseas Nationals)
12 Orthodox
   (including: Greek Orthodox Archdiocese of Thyateira and Great Britain; Russian Orthodox Church; Armenian Orthodox Church; Ukrainian Orthodox Church; Other Orthodox churches)
13 Church in Wales

Extract from coding frame for coding the transcript of recordings made in a qualitative study relating to the use of questioning in a tape-recorded teaching session

4 Rhetorical question
5 Question from student

   5a Answered by teacher
   5b Response from teacher of question to probe further
   5c Answered by another student
   5d Not answered immediately but within three minutes
   5e Not answered at all

You can see from Table 6.1 that single codes are sometimes allocated to a number of characteristics ('other Protestant', for instance, are all coded 11). This may be because there are very few specific instances of each type in the **dataset**. It is also affected by your research question – you may specifically want to know something about members of the Church in Wales (code 13), perhaps because they had commissioned a study of the health needs of religious workers. Although codes seek to retain the original variable values, they may be combined into a small number of categories for some analyses. They can still be used in their original form for other analyses (as the series of 5a–e codes for questions from students show).

Social class is often coded for in medical research. Stevenson, a medical statistician in the General Register Office, devised the social class scheme in the early twentieth century. A major revision in 1921 produced the five-class scheme which emphasised 'skill'. It has been used widely for the analysis of infant and occupational mortality and fertility and for monitoring population health (Szreter, 1984). Activity 6.1 shows the limitations of an otherwise fruitful concept.

ACTIVITY 6.1

To code the answer to 'What is your job?' in order to identify a person's social class you might use categories derived from the Registrar-General's social class based on occupation.

  I Professional etc. occupations
 II Managerial and technical occupations
III Skilled occupations

   (N) Non-manual
   (M) Manual

IV Partly skilled occupations
 V Unskilled occupations

Or indeed you might use socio-economic groups, which are a measure of employment status (not 'skill' or 'social standing').

Supposing, however, the purpose of the investigation was to assess how doctors' family life was affected by the demands of the job. What criteria would you then want to use to code the answers?

Factors such as hours worked, and whether it entailed shift work or absences overnight, could affect family life. Simply asking about the doctor's occupation would not be enough – you would have to ask additional questions about the number of hours worked and at what times. You might choose to see if F1s' family life was affected more than that of consultants. If so, you would code for different medical statuses, and have codes for the different responses to questions, asking respondents to state how often they did shifts, the numbers of hours worked and whether they felt their job interfered with their family life.

For each code you construct as you read through your qualitative data you need to write a short definition (perhaps giving examples). When later on you find another example that you think is covered by an existing code, check that it does and that the definition previously given would apply to this second instance. If it does not fit then you can create a new code (again noting it down with its definition). Note that creating new codes will mean revisiting previously coded material to ensure it does not fit the new code better (it is an iterative process, that is, you return to the material and repeat the coding in the light of later data as your understanding deepens). When eventually there are many codes, it becomes useful to sort them into groups. If several codes represent types of something, move them together under the common theme. Either put them in a list of their own, or make them subcodes of a major code (theme). This coding frame can be used by you as well as by others, and assures some degree of consistency between coders and across time. You can see that coding is not a trivial task.

Open-ended questions on questionnaires or interview schedules also will need a coding frame. To prepare the coding frame for quantitative research you start by selecting a sample of respondents' materials likely to maximise the variety of responses. The quick review of all your data when you started will help you do this as you can put a sticky note (or otherwise annotate) on the front of questionnaires that made a lot of points in the answers. Make a note of each type of response, allocating it to a category group with a definition and example as described for qualitative coding. Revise and resort until a stable set of categories seems to have emerged, with only a few instances of apparently unclassifiable responses being found. Codes for keying might also be needed for closed-end questions unless the response choices were precoded (i.e. they have numbers or letters corresponding to each response choice). Even forms with only closed-end precoded questions may require additional coding. Sometimes multiple responses to a single item or written comments from the respondent or the interviewer create unanticipated data you do not want to lose.

The coding frame (as well as the actual coding) can be developed by a team of coders working collaboratively; this facilitates consistency in the use of codes and also ensures clear instructions are recorded.

Code (including double-checking) and enter data

You should use spreadsheets, databases or a statistical analysis program (e.g. Microsoft Excel, SPSS, PASW or EpiInfo) to organise quantitative data (see the end of this chapter for further reading on how to use these programs). You should enter all of the data in the same format and in the same database to avoid confusion and difficulty with the statistical analysis later on. Lay out the data entry matrix in the same order as the questions on the questionnaire or interview schedule. Once you've entered the data it is crucial to check for accuracy. Although spot-checking a random assortment of participant data groups can accomplish this, it is not as effective as re-entering the data a second time and searching for discrepancies. This method is particularly easy to do when using numerical data because the researcher can simply use the database program to sum the columns of the spreadsheet and then look for differences in the totals.

Computer software to help with qualitative data analysis (QDA – NVivo or NUD*IST for example) helps both to store and retrieve data. The investigator still has to prepare, enter (or import), analyse and interpret text though. Software may call for special formatting or file structure and have file size or text line limitations, so this must be taken into account when preparing transcripts. Inadequately prepared transcripts from audio or digital recordings seriously delay qualitative data analysis.

Do record decisions taken about data preparation such as why something was given a particular code so that the rule can be applied consistently over time. It's surprisingly easy to forget the basis for a decision otherwise. Also you should plan how to track and store audio-taped and other materials. Rules for handling confidential or sensitive information (such as patient information) should be known by all involved in the coding process. Criteria for assessing the reliability and validity of transcripts need to be clear (for instance, do two people work independently to code up all the data, or is there a threshold number of transcripts where, if agreement is consistent between the two people, only a sample of transcripts is double-coded to ensure quality is maintained?).

Analysis of qualitative data is an iterative process. Atkinson and Heritage (1984) stressed that the production and use of transcripts are 'research activities'. They should not be treated merely as a 'technical detail' preceding analysis. Table 5.2 in Chapter 5 illustrates the point that transcription should retain the information you need from the verbal account for the methodology you have adopted. Field notes do not need to record overlaps and verbal hesitations, but a transcript for discourse analysis does.

It should be 'true' to its original nature. Added punctuation can alter the meaning of data. For example, hear the difference between:

1. 'I hate it, you know. I do'

and

2. 'I hate it. You know I do' (Poland, 2002, p632).

Listening to (copies of) interview tapes as you are transcribing and coding will help you with this. Transcripts should be double-spaced and have a wide margin to permit coding. Always work on an electronic copy of the original transcript so you know that the original is preserved intact. Back up your work regularly and store it securely, keeping originals of everything in a different place. With paper documents, take photocopies to code on.

Give each version of the copied transcript that you work on a sensible file name, and date it so there is an audit trail. It is usual to refer to the whole body of data collected as the **data corpus** and then the sample you select for scrutiny for a particular purpose is called the 'data set'. Months of structured observations of water contact behaviour, field notes, maps and interview transcripts formed the data corpus for a study of schistosomiasis transmission in Sudan. Yet the first data set to be examined related to excretion-related behaviour (Cheesmond and Fenwick, 1981). The reasons for this were because there was no previous published research on this, and because it was relatively quick to code up. On that occasion coding was done using coloured pencils (each activity had a different colour) and data were tallied on paper for analysis. Low-tech methods are still useful for analysing small amounts of data.

The basic coding process in qualitative research organises large quantities of text into much fewer content categories (also known as themes or nodes). Categories are patterns or themes that are directly expressed in the text or are derived from them through analysis. After that, relationships among categories are identified.

What you do when you code is provide boxes (categories) to hold the data. This classification enables you to measure the frequency of events and to examine how they relate to other events. Whilst some things can only be named (classified) and thus can only be counted, other things have properties that can be measured. This is addressed in the following two sections.

Why do we classify?

The purpose of classifying is to distinguish between variables that behave differently in terms of the problem being investigated. 'Variables' represent the constructs or the factors being studied. They summarise and reduce data in an attempt to represent the information needed to answer the research question.

If you were interested to explain completion rates amongst university students you would want to break down that very general category into a number of different variables (age, sex, degree registered for) but you might choose to ignore other possible categories (sport played, favourite food) because you think they are not relevant. Categories should be exhaustive (everything should fit somewhere) and mutually exclusive. In categorising there is a tension between retaining important distinctions in the data while seeking clarity and economy. In aiming for the fewest number of categories you do not want to be clumping dissimilar parts together. One way to approach this is to start with a few broad categories and then break them down into finer, more detailed ones.

It is easy to apply relevant categories used in everyday life – sex, age, marital status and occupation are examples. Sometimes, however, the categories arise either from the data or are theoretical concepts imposed by the investigator. You have taken people's height and weight measurements but what you want to examine is obesity (which means combining these measurements to create a new variable that is the body mass index). You then have to decide the threshold that classifies an individual as 'obese'. Case definition is important in epidemiological studies: what constitutes an episode of diarrhoea, for instance? It is a good idea to use classifications that will enable your results to be compared with other studies. The use of occupation as a basis for measuring class was stimulated by its link to health measurements such as mortality, as demonstrated through many research studies.

Measurement and classification

The coding frame provides a guide to the aspects of the data that will be analysed. Your choice of analytic techniques depends upon the variable types represented in your data. These might be qualities, such as marital status, or quantities, like age or income. The process of analysis involves comparisons between different groups of cases (whether at different points in time or place or against a 'gold standard', as happens in a clinical audit). To compare, one must assess, and measurement is one method of assessment. Activity 6.2 shows how variables that are qualities differ from quantitative variables with regard to the information they convey.

ACTIVITY 6.2

Thinking of your time at medical school:

1. Write down three quantitative methods of assessment you have experienced.
2. Write down three qualitative methods of assessment you have experienced.

You may have found it easier to think of quantitative methods like grades for an exam or passing a portfolio. The qualitative methods may not have come to you that easily but they are usually found as feedback, such as 'this assignment is satisfactory but it could be improved by doing this' or 'you'll make a caring doctor'. You probably felt you have a better sense of how much progress you are making with the quantitative assessment because of the scale that is used, as is discussed next.

Measuring and classifying quantitative data

Measuring quantitative data involves looking at certain variables. A variable is the name given to a category that can change its value. Quantitative variables may be ordinal, interval or ratio scales, whilst qualitative variables (that are simply a list of labels) are known as nominal variables. The level of sophistication of measurement increases for data measured by each level: nominal/ordinal/interval/ratio. These are explained below. If you use a lower measurement than is possible you lose available information, so it's preferable to use the highest possible level of measurement justified by the data.

The nominal level of measurement is the act of categorising (by types of mental illness or hobbies, for instance). Such categorical variables can be counted (the number of male or female students in a class) but cannot be ranked. You can report that there is a higher percentage of females in the medical school but that does not mean 'women are superior to men'. The **mode** (the most typical category) is the only statistic that can be used to summarise the average of a nominal distribution.

In ordinal scales cases are compared and if they are not equivalent then they are ranked. The Registrar-General's occupational class uses an ordinal scale. Among the dataset of an ordinal scale the appropriate average to use is the **median**. When cases are enumerated lowest to highest the median (average) is the middle case (where there is an odd number) or the midpoint between the two middle numbers if the total number of cases is even.

Interval and ratio are both metric scales where the interval between each class is the same. This means that arithmetic operations can be performed. Interval scales permit addition and subtraction while ratio scales also allow multiplication and division. The **mean** is the measure of central tendency average for both of them.

With interval scales, differences (intervals) between values are meaningful, but ratios of values are not. The values of the scores have meaning only in relation to each other. Temperature scales such as Fahrenheit and Celsius, and psychological scales for depression are examples of interval scales.

Ratio measurements possess a meaningful zero value. Physiological parameters such as blood pressure or cholesterol level are ratio measures. Mass, length and time are all ratio measurements used in scientific research.

Measuring and classifying qualitative data

In qualitative studies you will be coding data as you collect it and developing a coding frame as you go along. The evaluation or research questions you are trying to answer will suggest some categories, as may any relevant theoretical assumptions. If you are using qualitative software the use of memos to record the basis for your decisions can be tagged to the coded data; you will anyway want to write up a detailed coding framework as you code. Usually the memo about a code will include:

- the reason why you have created the code;
- a definition of what the code is about and the aspects the coded text reveals;
- why (and when) you have changed a code (for instance, if you renamed it);
- any ideas and questions about the analysis that occur to you as you code.

If you are working in a team and sharing the coding of the data, such memos are crucial. Colleagues know why you have coded the data in that way and such memos can be a starting point for further discussion. Reviewing these memos will help you later when you come to interpret your results.

The following case study, written in response to a request for an account for this book (thanks, Blanche and Michael) shows the practicalities of coding data and developing a coding frame.

Case study: Two medical students report their experience of developing a coding frame with qualitative data

Listening to transcriptions for the first time takes a bit of getting used to. It can be difficult to hear parts of the session, especially if there is a lot of background noise or over-talking. Also different accents, especially if you're not used to them, can make it more challenging. Listening to and understanding the audio is really important as the way something comes across is often largely dependent on small nuances of speech which you can't pick up on from the transcript alone. When listening to transcripts it is also difficult to not form opinions on the people you are listening to;

not having an opinion is obviously important for the neutrality of the research but it is surprisingly easy to do without realising.

The coding software itself isn't difficult to use and it's quite easy to pick up. To put it simply coding is like 'tagging' things on Facebook, you just select the piece of text you are referring to and attach the relevant code. When all the coding is complete, this enables you to search the software for different codes and you can see where things coincide or how codes are used in the text. What is more difficult is creating the codes. The idea behind creating codes is similar to creating a hypothesis in quantitative research. You need to think about what elements you would expect to make up what you are researching and then you create codes for each of these important elements, for example questioning is an important scaffolding technique so we created codes for each question type.

In order to create relevant codes it is important to discuss the different aspects and agree with the others involved as people can have very different views on what will occur. When the codes have been created it's important to remember codes aren't fixed, you created the codes based on what you think you might find, you might find you don't use them or you might find you need codes you don't have. If you need codes you hadn't originally thought of you can add codes though you don't want to end up with hundreds.

There are disadvantages of being involved in this kind of research. The coding itself is incredibly dull and repetitive, long hours of being sat at a computer which then only forms the basis of the analysis, so once the coding is finished there is still a lot to do. However, it is oddly rewarding and when you start to see patterns it does make it more worthwhile.

Blanche Lumb

A large part of my job was to code around 20 teaching sessions that had been audio-recorded and transcribed before analysing them. When I was actually carrying out the coding it was vitally important that the transcript was of sufficient quality to actually apply the codes, and since the people who transcribed my data were not medically qualified (and so were not familiar with some medical terminology) there were occasions where parts were mistranscribed. In some cases, there were transcription errors due to the poor quality of the recording, e.g. due to background noise, interruptions by other people or where participants spoke too quietly, too quickly or with strong accents. It was therefore useful when beginning to code a new session to listen to the whole recording once through *first alongside the transcription in order to spot and correct any areas that were transcribed incorrectly (disease and drug names were common errors!). This also allows you to get a feel for the people speaking (their voices, accents, knowledgeability, etc.) as well as to gain a rough idea of the structure of the session and the types of codes you are likely to use most often.*

As I was carrying out the coding it was also useful for me to be involved in creating and defining the coding framework myself so that I knew precisely what each code was to be used for. Making the definitions as explicit as possible and using examples of situations where a code could/could not be used makes the job much easier when it comes to applying them. Having definitions that are as detailed as possible also helps when there is more than one person carrying out the coding! When I first began coding I was often finding sections of talk that didn't fit neatly into the code categories I had created. One of the best ways I found to resolve these sections was to discuss them with other people, whether my supervisor or someone else in the office who could look at them with fresh eyes and give their own opinions on what they thought was happening.

I did however find that carrying out long sessions of coding requires continual concentration and became very demanding mentally. I found it was essential to take lots of short breaks in order to prevent myself becoming too tired and doing a poor job of it. There were also several occasions where sessions were actually quite uninteresting and yielded very little in terms of what I was investigating, meaning that coding these sessions was rather monotonous and unrewarding.

Michael Hollifield

Blanche and Michael's accounts make it clear how coding can be both boring and demanding. However, if it's your own research you will find that the drive to 'find out' spurs you on. Activity 6.3 shows you how researchers go about creating codes.

ACTIVITY 6.3

Go to Gibbs and Taylor's online qualitative data analysis site and listen to the three-minute clip where two Evidence for Policy and Practice Information and Coordinating (EPPI) Centre reviewers demonstrate the process of discussing a transcript and deciding upon themes and creating codes:

onlineqda.hud.ac.uk/Intro_QDA/how_what_to_code.php
www.methodspace.com/video/eppi-centre-and-ncb

In Activity 6.3 notice how the themes (categories) 'being bullied' and 'social isolation' arose out of the data through the process of intensively studying the transcript. 'Being bullied' was broken down further into 'physical abuse' and the 'consequences of being bullied'. A coding frame includes the process and rules for data analysis, thus making it systematic, logical and rigorous. The development of a good coding frame is the basis for being confident of the trustworthiness of research.

The success of analysis depends greatly on the coding process. You should do this systematically and stop for breaks when your mind starts to drift: it is most important that you are consistent and accurate. Careless entry of what represents the data will mean your analysis is worthless. Double-checking of randomly selected materials by a colleague working with you can help ensure quality control. It is this use of multiple coding that is addressed in 'What's the evidence?', below. Reliability relates to the consistency of a set of measurements or of a measuring tool (interview schedule, for example). Reliability is *necessary but not sufficient* for validity. In quantitative research interrater reliability is tested by giving two researchers the same thing to measure – they should agree. In qualitative research the use of two researchers to code the same transcript gives a similar assurance that the code is understood and consistently applied.

What's the evidence?

Multiple coding concerns the same issue as the quantitative equivalent 'interrater reliability' and is a response to the charge of subjectivity sometimes levelled at the process of qualitative data analysis. Although multiple coding does not usually demand complete replication of results, it does involve the cross checking of coding strategies and interpretation of data by independent researchers. While I would caution against multiple coding of entire datasets (on the grounds of economy in both cost and effort), some element of multiple coding can be a valuable strategy. It can be useful to have another person cast an eye over segments of data or emergent coding frameworks, and this is a core activity of supervision sessions and research team meetings.

Although six experienced researchers who independently coded one focus group transcript showed substantial agreement, Armstrong et al. (1997) found considerable variation in the ways that they packaged coding frameworks (including the language used). This is not surprising, given the complexity of qualitative data and the range of disciplinary backgrounds and interests of qualitative researchers. Indeed, Mauthner et al. (1998) have shown how researchers' original interpretations may shift when they revisit previously collected data.

However, the degree of concordance between researchers is not really important; what is ultimately of value is the content of disagreements and the insights that discussion can provide for refining coding frames. The greatest potential of multiple coding lies in its capacity to furnish alternative interpretations and thereby to act as the 'devil's advocate' implied in many of the

> Such exercises encourage thoroughness, both in interrogating the data at hand
> and in providing an account of how an analysis was developed. Whether this is
> carried out by a conscientious lone researcher, by a team, or by involving inde-
> pendent experts is immaterial: what matters is that a systematic process is
> followed and that this is rendered transparent in the written research project.
>
> (Barbour, 2001, p1116)

Having cleaned up your data and formed an overview of what you have, it is time to
move on to summarising your data. With quantitative data you need to learn about
the structure of your data, including identifying patterns, relationships or potential
anomalies, before you can select an appropriate statistical test for analysing your
data. You can do this by preparing graphs of the data, and calculating basic statistical quantities. Basic statistical quantities that should be calculated for the sample
dataset are the mean, standard deviation and median. Examining the minimum,
maximum and range of data can provide additional useful information. A frequency
plot (or a **histogram**) is a useful tool for examining the general shape of a data distribution (Figure 6.1).

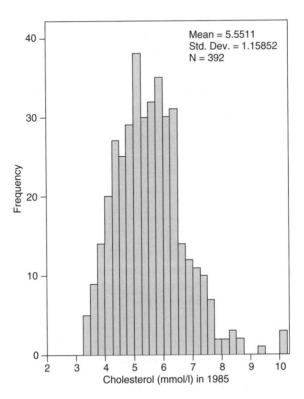

Figure 6.1 Example of a histogram (showing the distribution of serum cholesterol in a sample).

It graphically reveals any obvious departures from a normal distribution, such as skewness (a measure of the lack of symmetry in a distribution), in the data distribution. Non-parametric tests generally involve fewer assumptions about the underlying pattern of data distribution than their parametric equivalents. You should consult a statistician for the right statistical tests to use with the data distribution you have found. As part of this preparatory stage you should:

- make tables;
- inspect the number of responses to different questions (which may lead to decisions about combining categories);
- plan the analysis including, where relevant, statistical analysis such as correlations.

How to do this is discussed in this next section.

Summarising and displaying data

The next stage in data analysis is to reduce the materials collected so relevant patterns can be seen and you can then interpret what the data reveal. Analysis usually starts with descriptive analyses, to explore and get a 'feel' for the data. The analyst then turns to address specific questions based on the study aims or hypotheses, from findings and questions from studies reported in the literature and from patterns suggested by the descriptive analyses.

The choice of the most appropriate procedure for summarising and analysing the data is based on the preliminary data review you did before. Data reduction is a part of the analytic process and can be achieved through creating new variables, tabulation, coding, summarising, making clusters – anything that involves selection and focusing the data for a purpose. When creating new variables categories should be based on the nature of the phenomenon. For instance, a study of Down's syndrome might collapse all age categories to 'below 30 years' but a study of pregnancy rates needs a finer breakdown such as 20–24 years, 25–30 years, and even below 20 years.

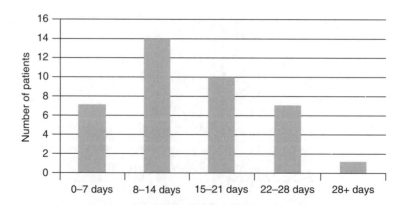

Figure 6.2 Bar chart showing average length of acute stay by patients admitted with a fracture of the neck of femur (average length of stay 14.64 days; range 2–29 days).

For statistical analysis in quantitative research the first step is to display and summarise data values. Using diagrams to display quantitative data makes it easier to interpret the data. If you are working with nominal or ordinal variables the bar chart (Figure 6.2) and the pie chart (Figure 6.3) are most useful. A histogram is used for interval/ratio variables.

Frequency tables are one form of basic analysis. These tables show the possible responses, the total number of respondents for each part and the percentages of respondents who selected each answer. Frequency tables are useful when a large number of response options are available, or the differences between the percentages of each option are small. In most cases, pie or bar charts are easier to work with than frequency tables.

Cross tabulations (cross tabs) are a good way to compare two data subgroups They let you compare data from two questions to determine if there is a relationship between them. Like frequency tables, cross tabs appear as a table of data showing answers to one question as a series of rows and answers to another question as a series of columns, as shown in Table 6.2.

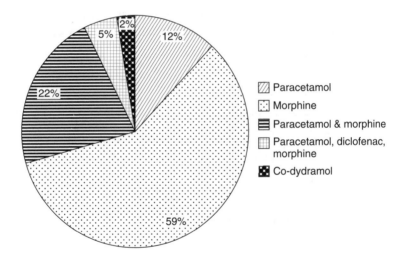

Figure 6.3 Pie chart showing the type of analgesia given to patients admitted with a fracture of the neck of femur.

Table 6.2 Cross tabulations

Person's role in the hospital	Female	Male
Doctor	50 (17%)	60 (29%)
Laboratory technician	40 (14%)	40 (19%)
Nurse	200 (69%)	50 (24.%)
Porter	—	60 (29%)
Total counts	290	210

Cross tabs are frequently used to look at answers to a question for comparing various demographic groups. The intersections of the various columns and rows (known as cells) are the numbers and percentages of people who answered each of the responses. In the example shown in Table 6.2 there is considerable gender disparity in nursing and porter roles. For analysis this is a great way to do comparisons.

Using tables, diagrams, maps, timelines and graphs helps you to see patterns that in turn suggest steps for further analysis. This is also a means of reducing the data to manageable proportions. Figures can display and summarise the broad characteristics of quantitative data, but it is easy to misrepresent data, so look out for this when appraising articles.

In giving talks or presentations, if a figure can represent the shape of the data or show relationships it communicates more effectively than tables. Dave Paradi has a very helpful website with a decision tree for selecting the best diagram to choose to display different types of results (**www.thinkoutsidetheslide.com/articles/using_graphs_and_tables.htm**; Figure 6.4). Essentially, aim to convey one message – whether it is to show proportion of parts (pie charts); how variables relate to each other (scatter plots, graphs, multiple box plots); data location, variability or symmetry (histograms, box plots or dot plots). Keep tables simple: several small ones are better than a large complex one. Tables work best when you want to show or compare precise values or where the values involve multiple units of measurement.

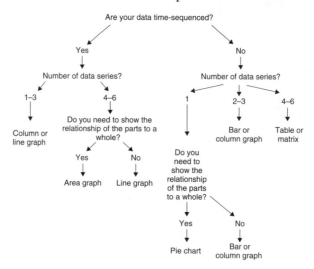

Figure 6.4 Flow chart for choosing an image to represent data (for a presentation or a report).

For figures make sure of the following.

- The caption title is self-explanatory (Who/what is depicted? From where? When were the data collected?). Usually the caption is set out underneath the figure, and the source is given. You may need to give footnotes or a key to explain.

- Axes on graphs are labelled clearly. The *y*-axis (upright) is used for the dependent variable; the *x*-axis (horizontal) is used for the independent variable.

- It's clear whether the scale is arithmetic or logarithmic.

- It's clear if there is a scale break (if the scale on the axes doesn't start at zero).

For tables make sure of the following.

- Titles are self-explanatory (Who/what is depicted? From where? When were the data collected?). The title should tell the reader what the table is about. The title goes on top of the table, and the source is given. Note that the date of a published source of data is usually different from the date given in the title (because of the lag between data collection and publication).

- The independent variables (if they have been identified) go in the left-hand columns, the dependent variables on the right.

- Rows and columns are clearly labelled.

- All abbreviations or codes are explained.

- There are row and column totals (although means/percentages may be more informative).

- Rows/columns are ordered logically (income or age in ascending or descending order).

- Numbers with decimal points are rounded to one or two effective digits (unless there is a good reason for greater precision). Numbers should always be right-justified in each cell.

- Sometimes it is better to put data into bands, e.g. <10 years, 10–15 years, 16–20 years. This makes the data more manageable, and easier to see trends and patterns.

Matrix construction is also useful in qualitative analysis. It is a systematic task that is also creative. It can help you to make sense of your data, so rather than think in terms 'Is this the right matrix?' your concern should be 'Is it helpful to me in thinking about my material?' Such a matrix could be used to tabulate specific observations recorded in a field diary by a researcher spending mornings with mothers with young children (Table 6.3).

Table 6.3 A matrix for tabulating qualitative data

Mother/child	*Mother's educational level*	*Excretion and hygiene response*
F1 / 4 months	2 years primary	Cleans child with edge of cloth wrap and kicks earth over faeces
F2 / 23 months	3 years primary	Tells child to use compost heap; dog follows to eat excrement and lick child's behind
F3 / 25 months	6 years primary	Tells child to use compost heap and to wash afterwards
F4 / 10 months	6 years primary	Guides child over potty and washes child and self with soap and water afterwards

Table 6.3 brings together material from extensive field notes that have recorded a variety of activities as they happened. Creating this matrix builds a picture that suggests a mother's educational status may be important for understanding hygiene practices in the home. Other observations suggest a particular role for dogs that could have relevance for the transmission of hydatid disease. Field notes would then be scrutinised carefully for observations that did not fit this pattern (that disconfirmed the emerging hypothesis). Activity 6.4 encourages you (alone or in a group if you prefer) to develop an observation matrix.

ACTIVITY 6.4

A group of you plan to audit hand-washing and the use of antiseptic gel in different wards in a hospital. It is decided that you will each take observations over a two-hour period at different times of the day over a seven-day period. Your method is structured observation.

Design an observational event matrix to display your observations.

A hand hygiene observation tool (HHOT) can be downloaded from **www.idrn. org/nosec.php**. The HHOT records hand hygiene opportunities, hand hygiene behaviours and the type of healthcare worker (HCW).

Hand-hygiene opportunities during patient care occur

(i) *before patient contact*
(ii) *after patient contact*
(iii) *after contact with patient's environment (space within curtains or patient's side room)*

Hand-hygiene opportunities are classified as

(i) *high risk (mucosa, body fluids, manipulating an indwelling device)*
(ii) *low risk (all other patient contact; contact with patient's environment)*
(iii) *unobserved level of risk (direct contact behind curtains)*

Hand-hygiene behaviours are classified as

(i) *alcohol hand rub (AHR) (use of AHR)*
(ii) *soap and water (use of soap and water)*
(iii) *no action (clearly observed to do neither)*
(iv) *unknown (no hand-hygiene behaviour seen before/after unobserved opportunity and AHR is behind curtains)*

HCWs are classified as

(i) *doctors*
(ii) *nurses (including healthcare assistants)*
(iii) *other/unsure (all others)*

(McAteer *et al.*, 2008, p225)

Having summarised your data (through developing themes, plotting graphs or tabulating results) you are now in a position to analyse your data.

Analysing data

Data analysis entails looking for points of similarity and points of divergence among the variables you haven chosen to collect or measure in order to answer your research question. Its aim is to describe facts, detect patterns, develop explanations and test hypotheses. Whether you have a quantitative, qualitative or mixed-method (**Q-squared**) study design, the depth of the analysis you are able to do will reflect how much time you have available. When deciding how you will analyse your data you may choose to do it manually using calculator, pen and paper or use a software program. The factors influencing your choice are:

- how much time is available for analysis;
- how long it will take you to learn and use a technique;
- the quantity of data you have collected (and its format);
- what training and support are available in your institution or elsewhere;
- the availability of equipment or software in your institution;
- what is the budget to pay for equipment or software and training (Basit, 2003).

With a mixed-method study design first analyse the study elements severally as outlined below – then integrate the findings from each to deepen understanding of the topic investigated.

Analysing quantitative data

Creating the cross tabs will show you the differences between variables relating to the topic of your research. For many studies this descriptive analysis is perfectly adequate and anyway needs to be done. You may draw up many more tables than you eventually choose to use when writing up: you only use those that are most interesting and relevant for your argument. However, you should never fail to report anything that does not support your argument.

For quantitative studies that are analytic in purpose you need to consider the appropriate statistics to use. This will depend on the type of variables you collected and you should refer to a statistics textbook. As was mentioned in Chapter 1, you always need to think about your data analysis when you are designing a quantitative investigation.

You will find it is useful to write down the thoughts that occur to you as you prepare tables. Seeing the patterns in data when you have collected the data yourself may spark additional questions or cast your thoughts back to the circumstances (and potential limitations) in which the data were collected. Recording these thoughts when they are fresh in your mind will help you reflect in a considered and nuanced way when you come to write up your material.

Analysing qualitative data

There are many approaches you could take to analyse qualitative data, but some are predetermined by your choice of methodology. For instance, for conversation analysis a preset list of phenomena that you would look for in your analysis stems from its theory (for instance, the knowledge of how breaking bad news is accomplished through the use of typical phrases, tone of voice and hesitations is grounded in the empirical observation and recording of that interaction). You are looking for the work that language does in constructing the meaning of an interaction. Other approaches, such as action theory or ethnography, put less restriction on your analytic approach. Thematic analysis is widely used to identify, analyse and report patterns (themes) within qualitative data.

The common features of analytic methods for qualitative research are:

1. Fixing codes to interview transcripts/field notes drawn from the data collection.

2. Making remarks of things that occur to you in the margin (or as memos in electronic files).

3. Sorting through materials to identify similar phrases, relationships between themes, common sequences and any distinct differences between subgroups.

4. Isolating patterns and processes, similarities and differences and pulling them out to be filed for the next stage of data collection.

5. Elaborating a small set of generalisations that cover the consistencies discerned in the data.

6. Confronting those generalisations with constructs or theories to build a formalised body of knowledge (Miles and Huberman, 1994).

In analysing qualitative data you constantly move back and forth between the entire dataset, the extracts of data that you have coded and the analysis of the data that you are producing (by way of themes). Writing is integral to analysis. It is not something that takes place last, as in the case of statistical analyses. Thus, start writing from the very outset. Note down ideas and potential coding schemes as data are collected and continue right through the entire coding/analysis process.

You should avoid the common errors in data analysis by:

- remaining flexible: be prepared to reassess your conclusions;

- understanding that some data are stronger than others and some sources are more reliable. If you collect the data yourself you will understand the context in which they were collected;

- looking for negative instances, finding out about outliers (the values at the extremes of distributions) and thinking about alternative explanations;

- understanding that missing data or data that are difficult to obtain may be important, so do not ignore them.

Whatever your approach to analysis, when you write it up it is vital that you explain what you did and why. If we do not know how people went about analysing their data, or what assumptions informed their analysis, it is hard to evaluate their research, let alone compare and synthesise it with other studies on the same topic.

You should write up results in the past tense. This also applies to what your respondents said or reported in any interview or questionnaire responses. Use of the past tense in this way avoids implying that:

- they may always hold those opinions;
- their opinions can be generalised to a wider population.

If you do want to make a generalisation (about human nature, for instance) then write it in the present tense.

Critical thinking

Whatever the form your analysis takes, you need to think critically when interpreting the data. This entails weighing up the evidence (in terms of its quality and the context in which it was constructed) to assess how far it supports or refutes your argument. Thinking analytically takes you beyond this point, in that you check for hidden assumptions, look for flaws in reasoning, weigh your ideas against those of others (and explain why different people came to different conclusions). You will draw on your personal experience with the relevant settings, respondents or documents to interpret your data, whether qualitative or quantitative. This is the topic of Chapter 7.

Chapter summary

- Data collection is not an end in itself – material needs to be prepared, summarised, displayed, analysed, interpreted, written up and presented to others.

- Before you start analysis, you need to prepare your data by checking, logging, entering or transcribing them.

- Coding is part of the analytic process in qualitative investigations.

- Coding frames help standardise the process and require careful construction.

- The purpose of classifying is to distinguish between parts that behave differently in terms of the problem being investigated.

- Summarising the data makes the data manageable and helps to identify patterns.

- Analysis requires you to be clear and consistent in your approach.

GOING FURTHER

Antaki, C (2002) An introductory tutorial in conversation analysis. **www-staff. lboro.ac.uk/~sscal/sitemenu.htm**.
A portal to very informative tutorials about this widely used form of discourse analysis.

Barbour, RS (2001) Checklists for improving rigour in qualitative research: a case of the tail wagging the dog? *British Medical Journal,* 322 (7294): 1115–17.
This article illustrates how rigour is assured in qualitative research.

Cohen, L, Manion, L and Morrison, K (2011) *Research Methods in Education,* 7th edition. Abingdon: Routledge.
This is a comprehensive textbook that is clearly written. It is supported by a companion website giving access to many useful additional learning materials.

Miles, MB and Huberman, AM (1994) *Qualitative Data Analysis: An expanded source-book,* 2nd edition. London: SAGE Publications.
An excellent and inspiring 'how to do it' book that includes ways to display data graphically.

Norušis, MJ (2011) *IBM SPSS Statistics 19 Guide to Data Analysis.* Upper Saddle River, NJ: Pearson.
This introduces the novice to both data analysis and the widely supported computing software SPSS and is supported by online materials/data CD-ROM. You'll learn how to describe data, test hypotheses and examine relationships.

Taylor, C and Gibbs, GR (2010) 'How and what to code'. **onlineqda.hud.ac.uk/ Intro_QDA/how_what_to_code.php.**
Many interesting video clips support the written information about how investigators can set about coding qualitative data. There are also useful tutorial materials and exercises.

Woods, D and Dempster, P (2010) Tales from the bleeding edge: the qualitative analysis of complex video data using Transana. **www.transana. org/support/CuttingEdge2010/.**
A 45-minute presentation from the Kwalon 2010 conference on 22 April 2010. It explores two projects analysing video data. The first ten minutes relate a project about childhood cancer that engaged with parents/hospital staff in 'grabbing the interesting clips and putting them into categories' (a 'hands-on form of coding'). The remainder (analysing a child playing video games) shows how multiple transcripts and screen shots can 'have complex data up and running at once to make sense of fast moving complex data'.

chapter 7

Interpreting the Implications of Research
Ann K. Allen

Achieving your medical degree

This chapter will help you to begin to meet the following requirements of *Tomorrow's Doctors* (General Medical Council, 2009).

Outcomes 1 – The doctor as a scholar and a scientist

12. Apply scientific method and approaches to medical research.

Outcomes 2 – The doctor as a practitioner

19. Use information effectively in a medical context.

The chapter will also enable you to meet the UK Foundation Curriculum (Academy of Medical Royal Colleges, 2012) requirements for engaging in and understanding research, audit and evaluation.

Chapter overview

After reading this chapter you will be able to:

- explain the difference between analysis and interpretation;
- evaluate the broader implications of research;
- interpret graphs, tables and other ways of representing data visually;
- apply research findings to clinical decision-making.

Introduction

Chapter 6 showed how data analysis is a critical, reflective and creative process. You alternate between data (its quality and 'shape'), the underpinning research question(s) and the theoretical paradigm. The next step is to make sense of your results by interpreting them in the light of what actually happened during data collection and the decisions you took while analysing the data. You also need to draw on what is already known about the topic in order to show how what you have found out confirms or challenges others' research and what it means for clinical practice. This is the final stage of the research process before you write it up or tell others about it. In this chapter we first explore what is meant by 'interpretation' and then go on to see how to interpret results. After considering how research findings can be applied to clinical practice the chapter concludes with an overview of how this happens.

You are perhaps wondering how data analysis differs from interpretation – and that is a good question to ask if you have been doing a qualitative study where everything seems to be woven together. However, if people didn't interpret their data they could end up describing what they wished they had found rather than what the data actually show. Our natural inclination with our own data is to assume that differences we see are real, and to minimise the contribution made by random variability (**Type I error**). Statistical hypothesis testing can help prevent you from making this mistake with quantitative data. If analysis concludes there is 'no statistically significant difference', you should not necessarily conclude that the treatment was ineffective. Quite possibly the study missed a real effect because you used too small a sample or your data were very variable. Obtaining a 'not significant' result when in fact there is a difference is known as a **Type II error**. When interpreting the results of an experiment finding no significant difference, you need to ask yourself how much power the study had to find various hypothetical differences if they existed. The power depends on the sample size and amount of variation within the groups, where variation is quantified by the standard deviation (SD).

You'll find that results are often equivocal because for various reasons you didn't collect all the data you wanted: respondents failed to reply or withdrew their consent; answers proved to lack detail or were ambiguous; organisational changes meant the study closed before the anticipated date so there were fewer respondents than the study needed to have the power to give meaningful results. How then do you make valid sense of what you actually have? This is the topic for the next section.

What is interpretation?

Data do not 'speak for themselves' – you, the researcher must first ask relevant questions of the data. Exploring quantitative data through descriptive and inferential statistics or qualitative data through coding and looking for relevant themes (as described in Chapter 6) only becomes meaningful when the analyst has an answer to find. Analysis involves exploring data to uncover trends and patterns such as relationships among different variables.

Data interpretation, on the other hand, means explaining the trends, patterns and relationships that emerged in the analysis. Because researchers interpret their findings in the context of their own knowledge and experience it is quite likely that two researchers with different backgrounds could interpret the same dataset differently. Which version is taken up by others will depend on a variety of factors, including what seems more plausible, useful or acceptable.

Interpretation involves:

- summarising and explaining the results of data analyses;
- relating the results to what is already known by comparing with similar studies

and looking back at the methods sections;

- evaluating the quality of the data – could mere chance explain what is observed?
- making sense of your data and realising what other information you need to explain what you have found and what else you wish you had looked for.

If you have ever written up a piece of research you may have seen comments on your work such as 'not relevant in the results section – put this paragraph in the discussion'. You are being asked to distinguish between 'the facts' (the results) and your opinion (explanation or interpretation) of those facts in the light of theory or of what is already known about this topic in the literature. If you are writing up your research as an article or as a dissertation this explanation or interpretation should come in the discussion section or chapter at the end.

Do beware of extrapolating findings outside the relevant population (or making claims unsupported by the evidence). The results of your study on the healthcare needs of Caucasian elderly residents of a suburban community (whom you accessed via Age UK) may not apply to an inner-city population of elderly people from minority ethnic groups. Although it is probably true for both groups that bereavement features heavily in their lives, they may hold very different responses to it. So do not suggest that 'what all elderly people need for support when they lose their partner is …' but instead relate your recommendations to the group you studied. It's quite reasonable to express the opinion that what you have shown might apply more widely, but do not treat it as an established 'fact'.

The research referenced below reports the investigation of the effect of clamping the umbilical cord at birth on neonatal anaemia in Sweden. The assertion is that delayed clamping reduces neonatal anaemia and improves iron status (perhaps by prolonging maternal perfusion). This would, of course, be protective in low-income countries where neonatal anaemia is prevalent. Activity 7.1 will give you some helpful pointers for writing up your discussion (Chapter 8). It also shows that researchers

---

ACTIVITY 7.1

The following study in Sweden was undertaken because many of the previous studies that informed a Cochrane review on the subject in 2007 were based in low-income countries where there was a high prevalence of infant anaemia. How far delaying the clamping of the umbilical cord would be relevant in more developed countries was thus questioned.

Andersson, O, Hellström-Westas, L, Andersson, D and Domellöf, M (2011) Effect of delayed versus early umbilical cord clamping on neonatal outcomes and iron status at 4 months: a randomised controlled trial. *British Medical Journal* 343: d7157.

Read the above article, paying particular attention to what is included in the discussion section.

take seriously the extent to which research findings can be extrapolated to other settings.

If you read the article in Activity 7.1 you will have noted that the structure of the discussion section is very clear. It contains:

1. a brief summary of the key findings;

2. a discussion of the strengths and limitations of the research process;

3. a comparison with other studies (including observation of an unexpected difference, giving a tentative explanation);

4. an interpretation of results (which includes linkages to the findings from other studies) and inferences drawn from them and this particular study;

5. a conclusion with a recommendation for future research.

This is a good structure to adopt with your own analysis of your research and when

---

Key questions in interpreting results

1. How good are the data?
2. Could chance or bias explain the results?
3. How do the results compare with those from other studies?
4. What theories or mechanisms might account for the findings?
5. What new hypotheses are suggested?
6. What are the next research steps?
7. What are the clinical and policy implications?

(Schoenbach, 2004, p482)

---

writing this up in your discussion. The box below summarises the key questions that you might try to answer when interpreting your results.

Research can be defined as *systematic and focused enquiry seeking truths that are transferable beyond the setting in which they were generated* (Greenhalgh, 2010, p189). Where newborn infants do not need resuscitation, the advantage of delayed umbilical cord clamping in the third stage of labour is to improve their iron status and reduce the prevalence of anaemia and iron deficiency at four months of age. In the UK it is not routine to delay cord clamping in full-term neonates, although there is increasing recognition in the midwifery and medical professions about its potential benefits, and if the mother expresses a desire for this it is facilitated. Andersson *et al.* (2011) stress that it is important to explore further the long-term effects of delayed and early cord clamping on health because there is no evidence whether infants deprived of placental blood have poorer neurodevelopment than those who receive placental transfusion. Godlee's editorial (2011) found the evidence of Andersson *et al.*'s research sufficiently compelling for her to recommend a change in practice (although she did not elaborate on why she found it compelling).

Students often comment on how frequently studies conclude with recommendations for further research. This recommendation is not a mantra to keep researchers employed. It stems from the nature of science itself. Research is a process whereby we come to know something more about the natural and social worlds. Through testing hypotheses against carefully collected and recorded data (from experiments or observations) we learn about 'what exists' and how it interrelates with other 'things that exist'. When hypotheses are refuted we seek explanations that are themselves testable in turn. Alternatively researchers clarify constructs and build theory through careful observation and induction that is tested against the data. Research proceeds painstakingly step by step with each new insight casting a beam towards fresh possibilities. Knowing the next step to take is a product of data interpretation, to which we now turn.

How do you interpret your data?

Interpreting your data (results) involves recognising and describing patterns or trends, or comparing an object or process to a standard (in the case of a clinical audit). Interpreting your results means determining the meaning and significance of the information against the questions posed in the research. It is the process of assigning meaning to the collected data and determining the conclusions, significance and implications of the findings. The process of interpretation will be affected by contextual information such as wider political, social and policy considerations as well as by the assumptions on which the questions were originally based.

Looking at your data (results) entails doing the following.

1. Consider how the data were affected by the context in which they were collected: are there any possible biases (from sampling, observer or instrument effects, for example)?

2. Identify the key results.

3. Consider alternative plausible explanations while you are selecting which one seems to 'fit best'.

4. Ensure you have a coherent argument that both explains your results and shows how they are relevant.

5. Ensure you have chosen the best method of presenting your results.

6. Identify a few feasible recommendations that follow on from your argument.

When you first started data analysis you will have looked at what you collected with a critical eye: what is missing? Does this create a bias of any kind? (Bias is dealt with in Chapter 3.) Statistical analysis is done to make inferences about the population from which the sample was drawn. This only works if a random sample was taken (so if you took a convenience or quota sample you must be realistic about what you can infer from it). Confidence intervals give a plausible range for the parameter of interest in the population: large samples make this range narrower so you can be more certain of the 'true' value.

> *Confidence intervals provide a statement about the precision of an estimate or esti-mates based on the amount of data available for the estimate. If a 'significant' associa-tion was not observed, then the confidence interval can give some idea of how strong an association might nevertheless exist but, due to the luck of the draw, not be observed.*
>
> (Schoenbach, 2004, p478)

However, do remember that something may be clinically significant without being statistically significant, and vice versa.

Figures or tables?

Patterns within large quantities of measurements are difficult to discern when laid out in tabular form. Graphs help researchers to interpret their data. When making sense of any graph there is a logical sequence of steps to follow.

1. Describe the graph. (What does the title say? What is on the *x*-axis (the bottom line)? What is on the *y*-axis (the vertical side line)? What are the units?)

2. Describe the data. (What is the numerical range of the data? What kinds of patterns can you see in the data?). Describing a trend based on information in a graph, you will notice how the amounts increase or decrease over the time period shown.

3. Interpret the data. (How do the patterns you see in the graph relate to other things you know?)

Look at Figure 7.1. The aim of the study from which this figure is taken was to deter-

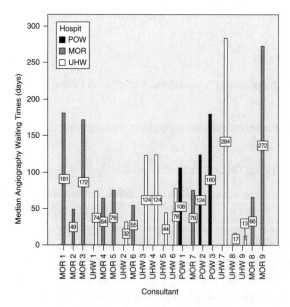

Figure 7.1 Graph of median angiography waiting times for various consultants.

mine whether three hospitals in South Wales were meeting the National Service Framework (NSF) for Wales 2004/2005 target of 80% compliance with a three-month waiting time for an angiogram, after referral by a consultant cardiologist.

The caption of this figure, taken from a student audit report, is not fully informative. It would be better as: 'The median angiography waiting times for the patients of 21 consultants in three hospitals in South Wales in 2005'. Consultant identifiers and their hospital are listed on the *x*-axis and the median average waiting times for an angiogram measured in days are shown on the *y*-axis. The logic of ordering the bars is not apparent – it would be more useful to cluster the bars representing consultants from each hospital together. Nor is it clear what happened with UHW8.

The range of 13–294 days shows considerable disparity between the different consultants within and between the three hospitals. In interpreting these results it's important to recognise the local differences between the hospitals (their size and role and service history) which affect the number of cardiologists employed and thus the number of angiograms that could be performed. Moreover, *The study did not determine the number of referrals each hospital received in this time and the number of those referrals which required an angiogram.*

The students very pertinently stated in interpreting their results that:

it is possible that the overall waiting time between being referred by the GP and having an angiogram is the same in all the hospitals over all. This could be because whilst patients at one hospital only wait three months for their angiogram after seeing a consultant, they may be waiting much longer for their initial consultation with the cardiologist than patients visiting another hospital. This may be due to manipulation of the lists so that patients intentionally wait longer for the consultant appointment, but the waiting time from consultant appointment to angiogram is within a reasonable time scale. This cannot be determined well from the study performed and would be useful to incorporate into future studies, as this clearly has implications for the results and how the results are used to view current waiting times.

ACTIVITY 7.2

Watch the short presentation on how to read and interpret different types of graph at: **www.youtube.com/watch?v=GA3RSbkcTzg** and compare this with the Open University Learning Space entry on interpreting graphs and charts: **openlearn. open.ac.uk/mod/oucontent/view.php?id=399402&section=5.1.**

Which did you find the more helpful – or were they about the same?

(MacDermott *et al.*, 2005, p19)

To take these steps further, do Activity 7.2, which offers other approaches to making sense of graphs.

The Open University site certainly reveals the various ways in which graphics can be used to mislead. Did you spot the difference in scales used in the first three graphs? Did you notice the use of numbers and ratios for presenting the data in the *Guardian* article? There's a clear message here that you really have to pay close attention. You may also find the links to other topics on this site useful if you feel daunted about the process of making sense of data. In presenting your own data you clearly want to select a means to make your argument convincing, but that does not involve misleading the reader.

By presenting data visually, complex datasets can be interpreted more easily. However, tables are needed so that other researchers can see the data that have been recorded: this ensures research is as objective as possible. As you saw in Chapter 6, tables can be used to present qualitative data but they are most frequently used to present numbers. It's much easier to read a table where numbers are neatly laid out in rows and columns than it is to make sense of a paragraph of sentences full of numbers. To be easy to read, tables should have a title and subheadings and ideally the source should be given. You'll recall that using percentages makes comparison between variables easy (as in frequency tables and cross tabulations). Be careful how you interpret them though. Look at the magnitude of the group – 10% of 500 is a great deal more than 10% of 5! This is why you should look for '$n =$' somewhere in the title of a table, and make sure you put it there too when you draw tables.

Table 7.1 is the kind of table you might see in an analytic study. Common statistical measures are expressed in it. An odds ratio is a measure of the strength of association between two binary variables. It is a descriptive statistic, where an odds ratio of 1 indicates that the condition or event under study is equally likely to occur in both groups. An **odds ratio** greater than 1 indicates that the condition or event is more likely to occur in the first group. An odds ratio less than 1 indicates that the condition or event is less likely to occur in the first group. It is possible that, unless

ACTIVITY 7.3

The following is taken from the paper: Morgan, O, McEvoy, M, Milne, L, Kumar, S, Murray, D, Man, W, Georgiou, M *et al.* (2007) Outbreak of *Salmonella enteritidis* phage type 13a: case-control investigation in Hertsmere, United Kingdom. *Euro-surveillance* 12 (7): E9–10.

A case control study was undertaken following an outbreak. Odds ratios were calculated for foods consumed at the event. The following table shows the results for eating an egg-mayonnaise bagel.

Table 7.1 Interpret a table

	Eaten	Case	Control	Odds Ratio	95% CI*	P-value
Egg-mayonnaise bagel	No	17	117	1.00		0.001
	Yes	32	11	19.5	7.9 to 51.7	

*CI = Confidence Interval

> If you were to interpret this table you would need to understand the meaning of these basic statistical concepts and explain their meaning for your results. The **null hypothesis** you will recall from Chapter 1 is a hypothesis that the researchers try to reject (nullify), because they believe it to be true. Remember that you can never prove a hypothesis but you can disprove it by testing it against the observed data.
>
> 1. What is the null hypothesis?
> 2. What does the odds ratio of 19.5 tell us?
> 3. Interpret the 95% confidence interval for the odds ratio.
> 4. What does a P-value of 0.001 tell us?

you are particularly interested, you may have skipped to the discussion section of papers where tables like this are interpreted for you. So if you haven't covered the relevant statistics (or epidemiology) yet, just notice how Table 7.1 in Activity 7.3 is laid out and have a go at interpreting what the numbers mean.

The question that the P-value answers is: if the populations to be compared really have the same mean overall, what is the probability that random sampling would lead to a difference between sample means as large (or larger) as you observed? As a researcher you are choosing either to believe in a coincidence or that the population means are really different. It is convention to use five times (or even one time) in a hundred as the threshold where you would believe a difference is more than a coincidence.

The answers are given at the end of this chapter.

Fallacies in research

Errors in reasoning can creep into the interpretation of data if there are unchallenged mistaken assumptions. A common one in epidemiological research is the **ecological fallacy**. This occurs when observations of relationships that hold for groups are assumed also to hold for individuals. So, for instance, whilst at population level a large waist (32 inches (81 cm) for women, 37 inches (94 cm) for men) is associated with increased risk of cancer, type 2 diabetes and heart disease, this is not necessarily true at the individual level. People have different shapes and heights. A World Health Organization (WHO) report (2011) showed there to be substantial evidence of sex and age variations in waist circumference and waist-to-hip ratio, and some evidence for ethnic differences.

In ecological studies the variables analysed are properties of localities, groups or populations, not individual people. An example is where the outcomes for patients who were hospitalised for acute myocardial infarction are compared between two countries in order to draw inferences about differences in the quality of care provided. Here individual data (patients' age and sex) are aggregated: mean age and sex ratios are calculated at the country level. In aggregating data information is lost, for instance ethnicity or social class. In such a study potential confounding factors (e.g.

type and severity of infarct or cardiac patient risk profile) that might also influence patient outcomes may not be available. Where a variable is related to both the outcome variable and to the exposure you are interested in, but is not a part of the causal pathway between them, it is known as a confounding variable.

You need to check for these sorts of errors when you are interpreting your data, and make sure you do not let them creep in when you come to write up.

Applying research findings in clinical practice

Healthcare professionals should apply their general medical knowledge and clinical judgement (their 'know-how') to assess the extent to which research-based recommendations apply in specific contexts. In deciding if evidence applies to a question you have about a patient, you saw in Chapter 2 that there are a number of points to consider:

- Is my patient so different from those in the study that results cannot be applied?

- What are my patient's likely benefits and harms from the therapy?

- How will my patient's values influence the decision?

- Is the treatment feasible in my setting?

When deciding what to do the first port of call is to look for available **guidelines** such as those produced by the National Institute for Health and Clinical Evidence or the University of York's Centre for Review and Dissemination. Websites of professional bodies (e.g. a relevant specialist site such as the Royal College of Obstetricians and Gynaecologists) may also be helpful. Where no such guidelines are available, search to see if there is a systematic review available on the Cochrane database and how recently it has been updated. Look for primary research (on PubMed, for example) only if no systematic review has been undertaken. The least reliable source (because it may be biased) is to sound out a local person claiming expertise. As this is the route for information most often taken, doctors need to keep their professional knowledge up to date. 'Googling' is only helpful if you use trustworthy sites that are both credible and recently updated.

If your research was a clinical audit or a health service evaluation then you will see in Chapters 9 and 10 how to ensure that your findings are translated into recommendations that are realistic enough to be speedily adopted. One dimension of interpretation here is to try to anticipate how the results might be interpreted differently by different categories of staff and to represent these objectively. To ensure the interpretation of results is as meaningful and unbiased as possible, you should review the results with internal colleagues and project or programme staff before finalising the evaluation report. This can be done by circulating an interim or draft report and holding a meeting to discuss it. That means the researchers will gain additional perspective on the meaning of the data from the reviewers before writing the final draft. Discussions with others can also add to the rigour of the final document and build consensus about the recommendations to improve clinical practice.

Although not labelled as research, your elective experience has many of the characteristics of a research project. You started with aims and learning objectives (that may have changed in the light of reality) and for most people it can be a transformative experience as they come to make sense of (interpret) what they have learned (the results). For instance, a student, Holly Jacques, writes about an elective in a poorly resourced country:

> *If I was to have another opportunity to experience medicine in a different setting I would try and contact the centre I was visiting earlier. This would have given me more time to discuss the range of diseases I would see and to allow me to carry out more in depth self directed learning into them before I left. I would also have liked to be able to be of more assistance to the hospital. Although I took out books, on arrival I realised they were also desperately short of basic equipment such as stethoscopes. If I was to visit again I would have spent time fund-raising and organising this equipment. As it is since returning home I have asked for a list of needed equipment and further books so I can hopefully send further aid to the hospital.*

This reflection is an interpretation of the results of participant observation in a very different clinical setting.

Mainstreaming research in policy-making

The previous section mentioned guidelines. These and NSFs represent research that has been **mainstreamed** into practice. To make a difference, research needs to influence policy and practice. This is both a political and a cultural issue. Since the 1960s there has been a drive to influence decision-makers through what is now known as evidence-based policy. Politicians in democracies work to short timeframes – their interest is in being re-elected. Social or religious attitudes can inhibit research results from being acted on, especially in sensitive fields such as reproductive health or HIV/AIDS. In particular, low-income countries may lack the capacity to make use of research advances (although initiatives such as the global network Healthcare Information for All by 2015 seeks to address this: **www.hifa2015.org**).

Diversity of opinion is the life blood of scientific research: researchers know that it is not always possible to resolve important controversies. Yet this scientific uncertainty and debate can seem in the popular imagination to undermine the credibility of discovery. Breakthroughs are rare: they are the result of small steps steadily and systematically made. The careful evaluation of results takes time, and the length of time from discovery to developed application is more probably a decade rather than days. Researchers of all kinds speak a different language from policy-makers, and have very different interests. Education about the value of research is needed at all levels. As Cochrane advocated, *statistically astute surveillance* is relevant to health systems globally (Cochrane and Blythe, 1989, p177) and this is why epidemiology and statistics are a vital component in medical education. Growth of translational research and **implementation research** reveals how organisations can bridge cultural divides, as was shown in Chapter 1.

Under conditions of uncertainty, policy-makers turn to researchers for advice. The very complexity of clinical problems often requires global networks of researchers to link their expertise. Such **epistemic communities** (Haas, 1992) comprising scientists with experience of working for different organisations – universities, pharma and WHO – have mobilised global action through the United Nations system in recent planning for a possible influenza pandemic (2005). Governments were encouraged to adopt the template pandemic flu plan developed by WHO, adapting it to suit local circumstances. Meetings were held in all continents to raise both awareness and resources.

As a medical student, these organisations and processes may seem a little remote from your own world unless, of course, you belong to Medsin (**www.medsin.org**), which adds the medical student's voice to international advocacy. Medsin was responsible for putting global health outcomes into *Tomorrow's Doctors* (General Medical Council, 2009). As you read earlier in the elective student's quotation, with preparation there are ways for medical students to contribute to improving global

---

ACTIVITY 7.4

Find out what plans are operational in your medical school if there is a global pandemic. Is information easily found on your university's web page? How would a flu pandemic affect medical students? Have you discovered anything that might be improved?

---

health.

The threat of pandemic flu remains ever present. Activity 7.4 asks you to research how the WHO suggestions have been implemented in your medical school and to reflect on how what is proposed might be improved. The purpose for 'finding out' should be to guide future action.

If you found this information either difficult to locate or not recently updated you might think of various explanations – in doing that you will be interpreting the data you found in the light of your knowledge about the local context of your medical school. The next section outlines specific ways in which research is feeding through into practice.

Looking at the wider implications of research

Case study: How genetic advances sparked by the Human Genome Project (HGP) may affect the practice of medicine

All diseases have a genetic component, whether inherited or resulting from the body's response to environmental stresses like viruses or toxins. The successes of the HGP have even enabled researchers to pinpoint errors in genes – the smallest units of heredity – that cause or contribute to disease.

The ultimate goal is to use this information to develop new ways to treat, cure, or even prevent the thousands of diseases that afflict humankind. But the road from gene identification to effective treatments is long and fraught with challenges. In the meantime, biotechnology companies are racing ahead with commercialization by designing diagnostic tests to detect errant genes in people suspected of having particular diseases or of being at risk for developing them.

An increasing number of gene tests are becoming available commercially, although the scientific community continues to debate the best way to deliver them to the public and medical communities that are often unaware of their scientific and social implications...

Disease intervention

Explorations into the function of each human gene – a major challenge extending far into the 21st century – will shed light on how faulty genes play a role in disease causation. With this knowledge, commercial efforts are shifting away from diagnostics and toward developing a new generation of therapeutics based on genes. Drug design is being revolutionized as researchers create new classes of medicines based on a reasoned approach to the use of information on gene sequence and protein structure function rather than the traditional trial-and-error method. Drugs targeted to specific sites in the body promise to have fewer side effects than many of today's medicines.

The potential for using genes themselves to treat disease – gene therapy – is the most exciting application of DNA science. It has captured the imaginations of the public and the biomedical community for good reason. This rapidly developing field holds great potential for treating or even curing genetic and acquired diseases, using normal genes to replace or supplement a defective gene or to bolster immunity to disease (e.g., by adding a gene that suppresses tumor growth).

(US Department of Energy Genome Programs:
**genomics.energy.gov. www.ornl.gov/sci/techresources/Human_
Genome/medicine/medicine.shtml**)

Research arises out of, and has implications for, the setting in which it occurs, but may have much wider implications if it leads to opportunities to change the approach to practising clinical medicine fundamentally, as this case study of genomics describes.

Progress is driven partly by commercial opportunities but, as noted, social and legal systems may lag behind where people are unaware of potential consequences of genetic testing. Insurance companies build estimates for their premiums on the basis of shared risk. Genetic tests make it potentially possible to discriminate between people who have a greater risk of developing a disease than others. It may be that some people will not find themselves able to take out a life insurance policy to protect their dependants, just as people living in the flood plains of rivers find it difficult to get affordable building and home insurance in some parts of the UK.

Genomics' potential for therapeutic interventions is commercially and clinically attractive and the field is fast-moving. However, 'big picture research' addressing a clinical problem is not always translated into action very quickly, as earlier chapters have shown (it was half a century before the Navy provided lemons to prevent scurvy in their sailors, for instance). There is still debate about the use of low-dose aspirin in the primary prevention of vascular disease (Antithrombotic Trialists' Collaboration, 2009). The risks of serious bleeds might outweigh the beneficial effects of reducing the risks of stroke or coronary heart disease, so further trials are being conducted.

Practitioners, through audit and local small-scale research to improve the quality and safety of healthcare, potentially have both the opportunity and the motivation to change practice (see Chapters 9 and 10). However, large-scale and complex changes, even if politically desired and clinically approved in principle, can suffer delays for a variety of reasons. Summary care records (SCRs) are intended for use in emergency and unscheduled care in England. They are held on a national database over a secure internet connection to be accessible to authorised staff in the English NHS. Drawn from the electronic record held by a person's GP, they comprise three data fields – medication, allergies and adverse reactions. The introduction of SCRs in England from 2007 started slowly even among primary care trusts that were early adopters (Greenhalgh et al., 2010a). This was because some GP practices had ethical concerns relating to issues around patient confidentiality and securing informed consent; some practices lacked the resources to check the patient data that were to be input into the national database; or participation in the roll-out was rated low in their priorities so data transfer was put on the back burner.

In 'What's the evidence?' you can see some problems for interpreting results when evaluating complex organisations. One expected outcome of this mixed-method study was that access to SCRs would speed up consultations. In fact, the quantitative data showed that consultations were often longer when records were retrieved than when they were not. A possible confounding variable to explain that finding might be that where a patient had more than one complaint, or had a complex illness, the SCR was more likely to be sought. This was borne out by the ethnographic observations of clinical encounters.

Not everything that is relevant is measurable. The outcome 'improved patient satisfaction' could not be assessed because it's the whole consultation that affects how a patient feels, not just whether there is an SCR. Some clinical staff perceived the use of smart cards and passwords to access the data to be an irritating waste of time, particularly if they believed the data might not be accessible or could be inaccurate. It seems that in some settings it was culturally acceptable to leave the computer logged on while not attending to it (with the attendant risk of unauthorised access to patient data). Those responsible for maintaining data security were naturally concerned about that possibility. In secondary care settings such as accident and emergency, where multiple users need access to one computer, accessing SCRs becomes

What's the evidence? Evaluation of a nationally stored electronic Summary Care Record in England

The evaluation found: *The main determinant of SCR access was the identity of the clinician: individual clinicians accessed available SCRs between 0 and 84% of the time. When accessed, an SCR seemed to support better quality care and increase clinician confidence in some encounters. There was no direct evidence of improved safety, but findings were consistent with a rare but important positive impact on preventing medication errors* (Greenhalgh et al., 2010b). 'E-governance' refers to maintaining the security of access to electronically held confidential information.

> *... key characteristics of program success may not be articulated in the vocabulary of outcomes and may not yield to measurement. One such dimension of the SCR program was the variable culture of e-governance across different organisations (e.g., the extent to which it was acceptable for staff to forget their passwords or leave machines 'logged on' when going to lunch).*
>
> *Finally, program learning that leads away from initial objectives threatens failure against outcome criteria. In the SCR program, an early finding was that predefined milestones (e.g., number of records created by a target date) were sometimes counterproductive since implementation teams were required to push forward in the absence of full clinical and patient engagement, which sometimes led to strong local resistance. We recommended that these milestones be made locally negotiable. But because critics of the program interpreted missed milestones as evidence of 'failure', policymakers took little heed of this advice ...*
>
> *In the real world of eHealth implementation, designers design, managers manage, trainers train, clinicians deliver care, and auditors monitor performance; people exhibit particular personality traits, express emotions, enact power relationships, and generate and deal with conflict. Technologies also 'act' in their own non-human way: for example, they boot up, crash, transmit, compute, aggregate, and permit or deny access. A statistical approach may produce more or less valid and more or less reliable estimates of effect size (and hence a 'robust' evaluation), but 'When we enter the world of variables, we leave behind the ingredients that are needed to produce a story with the kind of substance and verisimilitude that can give a convincing basis for practical action'.*
>
> *The narrative form preferred by social scientists for reporting complex case studies allows tensions and ambiguities to be included as key findings, which may be preferable to expressing the 'main' findings as statistical relationships between variables and mentioning inconsistencies as a footnote or not at all. Our final SCR report was written as an extended narrative to capture the multiple conflicting framings and inherent tensions that neither we nor the program's architects could resolve.*
>
> (Greenhalgh and Russell, 2010)

more problematic.

The point is also made in this extract that to produce a convincing case for practical action (which is a major part of interpretation) the stories accounting for peo-

---

Chapter summary

In this chapter interpretation is explained as the process whereby you make sense of your data. It involves:

- explaining the results of the data analyses and considering certain key factors (such as data limitations and the context of the inquiry) when interpreting the data;

- relating the results to what is already known;

- suggesting new research possibilities or the broader implications of research findings.

We also explored:

- the role of research in generating new knowledge and the time this requires to put into practice;

- the social processes associated with putting research into practice, including clinical decision-making.

---

ple's different behaviours need to be told and understood.

Variation in criteria for success among different stakeholders reinforces the point made earlier, that when interpreting your data in any evaluation research you need to consider the different viewpoints held.

Answers to Activity 7.3

1. What is the null hypothesis?
   There is no difference in the proportion of cases and controls of those who ate egg-mayonnaise bagels.

2. What does the odds ratio of 19.5 tell us?
   Cases had 19.5 times the odds of having eaten egg-mayonnaise bagels than controls.

3. Interpret the 95% confidence interval for the odds ratio.
   We can be 95% certain that the true odds ratio lies somewhere between 7.9 and 51.7.

4. What does a *P*-value of 0.001 tell us?

The probability of observing this odds ratio (or larger) if the null hypothesis is true is 0.1%, which is very small, providing strong evidence to reject the null hypothesis.

Did you spot that the egg-mayonnaise bagels were implicated for causing *Salmonella enteritidis*?

GOING FURTHER

Bowling, A and Ebrahim, S (2005) *Handbook of Health Research Methods: Investigation, measurement and analysis.* Maidenhead: Open University Press.
A comprehensive overview of researching health that includes genetics and psychosocial biology.

Greenhalgh, T and Russell, J (2010) Why do evaluations of ehealth programs fail? An alternative set of guiding principles. *PLoS Medicine* 7 (11): e1000360.
Worth reading because it spells out the differences in the positivist and interpretivist paradigms (helpfully summarised in Table 1), and invites readers to add comments to the points made.

Schoenbach, VJ (2004) Data analysis and interpretation: concepts and techniques for managing, editing, analyzing and interpreting data from epidemiologic studies. **www.epidemiolog.net/evolving/DataAnalysis-and-interpretation.pdf**.
This chapter explains the process and issues clearly.

chapter 8

Communicating the Outcomes of Research and Evaluation

Ann K. Allen and Seema Biswas

Achieving your medical degree

This chapter will help you to begin to meet the following requirements of *Tomorrow's Doctors* (General Medical Council, 2009).

Outcomes 1 – The doctor as a scholar and a scientist

8. The graduate will be able to apply to medical practice biomedical scientific principles, method and knowledge.

   (g) Make accurate observations of clinical phenomena and appropriate critical analysis of clinical data.

9. Apply psychological principles, method and knowledge to medical practice.
10. Apply social science principles, method and knowledge to medical practice.
11. Apply to medical practice the principles, method and knowledge of population health and the improvement of health and healthcare.
12. Apply scientific method and approaches to medical research.

Outcomes 2 – The doctor as a practitioner

19. Use information effectively in a medical context.

    (c) Keep to the requirements of confidentiality and data protection legislation and codes of practice in all dealings with information.
    (d) Access information sources and use the information in relation to patient care, health promotion, giving advice and information to patients, and research and education.

Outcomes 3 – The doctor as a professional

20. The graduate will be able to behave according to ethical and legal principles.
21. Reflect, learn and teach others.

    (c) Continually and systematically reflect on practice and, whenever necessary, translate that reflection into action, using improvement techniques and audit appropriately – for example, by critically appraising the prescribing of others.

The chapter will also enable you to meet the UK Foundation Curriculum (Academy of Medical Royal Colleges, 2012) requirements for engaging in and understanding research, audit and evaluation.

Chapter overview

After reading this chapter you will be able to:

- identify the ethical responsibilities of authors;
- explain intellectual property and copyright;
- write up your findings clearly in an appropriately structured way;
- tell others about your findings through academic reports, at conferences, online or through publication in a peer-reviewed journal.

Introduction

It is now time to write up and possibly tell others about your research. Remember your original purpose. If it was to discover new knowledge you will be keen that not only should your academic report gain you a worthy mark, but others should know about it. If your investigation was to improve practice then others also should know what needs changing and why.

This chapter aims to help you complete the writing-up stage of your research successfully and consider the various ways you can disseminate your research. We start by reminding you about the ethical responsibilities of authors. You are probably aware about plagiarism but you may have thought about it as 'an academic rule' to trip up unwary students rather than an ethical issue relating to intellectual property rights. Writing for academic purposes is likely to be high on your agenda so that is dealt with first (along with creating posters and presenting at meetings). Wikis and blogs increasingly form part of communicating in academia and we encourage you to try these out (if you are not already doing so).

Then, because it will help you with getting your first Foundation post or later jobs, we look at how you go about getting your name into print, together with practical matters associated with that. Finally, it is very important for you to know about copyright, including what is meant by creative commons and moral rights, once you start to publish.

Ethical responsibilities of authors

As professionals, doctors are concerned to act with integrity, and this first section explains ground rules relevant to the dissemination of research (communicating your findings). As an investigator you conscientiously kept complete records of your findings, ideas and decisions. They were filed for ease of retrieval while being stored securely (e.g. with password protection of electronic files). In data analysis you looked for disconfirming cases and sought to explain them. Now you come to write up your findings it is important to ensure that all statements of fact are true, that there is evidence to support all of your assertions (or 'claims') and that you acknowledge others' ideas by proper citation and referencing.

Intellectual property

Whatever you create is your intellectual property. Authors, publishers and organisations own the documents or ideas they create and these are subject to national and international copyright laws. An organisation (such as a university) employing staff members who create original work may be the holder of the copyright for that work yet permit staff to publish or otherwise disseminate their own creations. Similarly, an assignment you produce for a university assignment may be copyrighted through the university. Copyright will be discussed later because it becomes relevant when you publish work. Plagiarism, which is an ethical rather than a legal matter, has to be avoided when you cite your sources and acknowledge quotations properly in your academic writing. Plagiarism is a serious academic offence and people have been stripped of their degrees and lost their reputations when such fraud is uncovered. The following extract in the 'What's the evidence?' box below explores the harmful nature of plagiarism.

What's the evidence? Plagiarism

One of the most insidious forms of plagiarism is unattributed use of material to which one has acquired confidential access in a review process. The academic grapevine bears stories of people who have plagiarized others' work that appeared in grant proposals or manuscripts under review. Such plagiarism can be difficult to prove when the original work is not only unpublished but secured under the provisions of confidentiality.

The U.S. Federal definition of plagiarism includes misappropriation of another's ideas. Ideas shared in hallway conversations or at research conferences (as, for example, in poster sessions) may seem fair game for competitive appropriation. If, however, a researcher knows that someone else appropriated the idea and used it without acknowledgement, the incident will seem more a matter of plagiarism than gamesmanship. It will, unfortunately, be difficult to prove, and so such cases are not usually investigated as misconduct.

Harmfulness of plagiarism

Authorship signifies both credit and responsibility for the processes and outcomes of research. Plagiarism breaks the connection between a researcher's ideas and the credit justly deserved for those ideas, but it also distorts the record as to who is responsible for those ideas. It introduces false information into the scientific system, which is fundamentally based on truth.

Plagiarism increases the strain on the system of research publication. Previous cases lead wary editors and reviewers to check not only the scientific value but also the originality of manuscripts and proposals submitted. Plagiarized findings that are republished more or less intact take up valuable publication space that could otherwise be used for original research. They also skew the research record by appearing to show further evidence of already published results, thereby distorting meta-analyses. Small changes that plagiarizers make to escape detection may also introduce errors or inaccuracies.

(Anderson and Steneck, 2011, pp91–2)

In addition to avoiding plagiarism, you need to be aware of how you use forms of media in your research. Whenever you use media such as photographs and drawings of human subjects, there are ethical issues involved. These include discrimination on the basis of sex or minority/racial groupings as well as privacy issues. Permission must be sought and given if such images are to be used, and the persons in them should be unrecognisable as individuals. Permission must be granted even if the photograph shows only someone's foot and its ulcer.

Different academic products

Reports (dissertations and theses) often form the final product of a degree because the student can demonstrate a wide range of knowledge and skills in them. Other work such as posters and presentations to submit at conferences may also be encouraged, along with communicating through blogs and wikis either as a part of course work or as an assessment of it. How to get the most from these is the topic of this section. We've giving writing for journals a section of its own because that form of writing has rather different ground rules.

Writing academic reports

Short essays and laboratory reports enabled you to demonstrate basic academic skills such as displaying knowledge of relevant conventions about the writing process as well as of the substantive area. However, they probably were quite short documents. If you are doing research as part of your programme you will probably be expected to write a research report or a research dissertation of several thousand words, which can feel quite daunting. However, once you break it down into its structural components and plan to write a section at a time you'll find it becomes simply a matter of starting – and keeping going. Incidentally, the process is helped if you plan to complete a section at a time – but if you are interrupted, do make sure you write the gist of what you were going to say next to help you pick up the flow when you return to it.

Different parts of an academic report (a dissertation or thesis) do different jobs – this is the meaning of 'structural components'. In writing an essay you learned to write a conclusion that provided a summary of the key points previously elaborated in paragraphs of your argument, and demonstrated how you answered the question. You learned that in an essay the conclusion (and the introduction) had special roles and were effectively each other's mirror images. In a dissertation or thesis, by convention every section (or chapter) has its own particular role that the reader expects will be complied with.

Activity 8.1 will help you write a coherent, logical and concise account that explains your data to an interested reader. There should be an analytic story reflecting your approach (the question and the theory) whether you were testing a hypothesis or seeking to build one. This means you go beyond simple description of the data to construct an argument in relation to your research question.

ACTIVITY 8.1

List the headings of your report in the order in which they will appear in the table of contents. Now number them in the order in which you think they will be written.

People rarely start writing at the beginning, marching forward to the end. They start with what's easiest to write. Some of you will have discovered that, with the exception of exams (and not always then) and even with a detailed plan, you tend to write a paragraph in one section, a few sentences in another and go back and forth as your thinking evolves with your reading and with discussions with your friends. Even though it may be much easier to write fluently if you know what you plan to argue and write a section at a time, we all have our own ways that work for us. People have different approaches to writing and a good way to learn is to talk to others about how they do it.

This process of creation is certainly made much easier with word processing. Drafting and redrafting scripts is normal practice, which is why it is recommended that you do not leave matters to the last minute but start writing early and write often. With a short essay it's possible for the material you've read to be held in your head to be distilled into an answer to the question. But now we are talking about writing up your investigation and there are several distinct aspects to it, such as why you did the study, how you did it, what were your results and what they mean. Activity 8.1 asked you to list report headings that would appear in the table of contents of a research report. Figure 8.1 illustrates a not-infrequently observed first attempt by many students (who probably have not gone to look for an example of a report and so are drawing on their general knowledge of books they've read).

Chapter 1 . . . . page 1
Chapter 2 . . . . . . page 12
Chapter 3 . . . . . . page 23
Chapter 4 . . . . . . page 32
Conclusion . . . . . page 41
Appendix . . . . page 49

List of tables and figures

Figure 8.1 A table of contents.

Figure 8.1 does not say much, beyond how many pages there are to read. But I have read reports that gave such (un)informative titles. There is a formalised structure for report writing that scientists writing up their research use (IMRAD). This mnemonic stands for introduction, methods, results and discussion. These will be looked at more closely in the next section. The principle is no different when you are a medical student from how it was at school. Someone who follows your method and repeats your work under the same conditions should be able to get the same results as you. You should only include material that is relevant to your argument. This gives your writing clarity. The account you are giving is about what you did and what you found. It's useful to ask your tutor if you can read examples of highly graded reports so you have a better idea of what is wanted.

Activity 8.1 also asked you to consider the order in which chapters are likely to be written – we shall turn to this now.

Stages of writing

The components of any piece of scientific writing placed in the order they appear in the table of contents are given below (with the order in which they are written in brackets). Each is discussed in more detail further on.

- title (7);
- abstract (8);
- introduction (6);
- methods (1);
- results (2);
- discussion (and recommendations) (5);
- reference list (3);
- appendices (4).

The numbers in brackets represent the usual order of writing the final draft. A clearly structured argument links the material in the introduction to the results and the discussion. The methods should be appropriate for the question identified (see Chapters 1 and 4) and data should be interpreted in the context not only of the background presented in the introduction but also the limitations of the methods used.

You cannot begin your research until you've decided on the methods so it makes sense to write these up as soon as possible. Then when you have the results they need to be analysed, so that is a major activity that will be written up as you do it. By the time that is done you will know what, if any, material needs to appear in the appendices (such as interview schedules so the reader knows what questions were asked). So this material can be written and filed away for later insertion.

Some would suggest writing the reference list after the discussion. But you will be reading literature and keeping records of everything you've found useful right from the start. Unlike in some other disciplines (and all postgraduate theses), it is not expected that there will be a separate chapter called 'literature review' – instead you are expected to integrate your reading wherever it is relevant, particularly in the discussion. By the time the discussion is written most of the references will already be tallied, and it's important not to leave the references to the last minute. Besides, it sometimes helps to break a writer's block to start (and add to) the list of references. Remember to delete any you decide not to use.

A report of a qualitative study may be less rigidly structured than this: the results and discussion are often, although not always, merged together or in a separate 'findings' section (see 'What's the evidence?').

What's the evidence?

This draws on an evaluation of the introduction of summary care records in England that was reported in Chapter 7. An interim report of a mixed-methods, longitudinal, multisite, sociotechnical case study to evaluate the implementation and adoption of detailed electronic health records in secondary care in England was published (Robertson *et al.*, 2010). This article in fact follows the IMRAD layout, but the results section (focusing on themes from the macroenvironment and cross-cutting themes particularly relevant to English health policy and debates about approaches to implementing electronic health records) is much longer and more discursive than you would find in a bioscience journal. The pdf version is 12 pages, which is long for a scientific journal. The online version makes use of the capabilities of the internet with hyperlinks to data supporting the identified themes.

We shall now look at each of the report components in turn.

The title

The title of your report should be concise and informative. It should encapsulate the essence of the research and should not be vague and general. To see how useful an informative title can be, try Activity 8.2.

ACTIVITY 8.2

Scan the table of contents of three different journal titles in your library.

Can you find examples of vague/general titles? If so, can you do better?

Examples of titles that I found self-explanatory include:

Greenhalgh, T, Stramer, K, Bratan, T, Byrne, E, Mohammad, Y, Russell, J (2008)

Introduction of shared electronic records: multi-site case study using diffusion of innovation theory. *British Medical Journal,* 337: a1786.

Schiff, GD, Bates, DW (2010) Can electronic clinical documentation help prevent diagnostic errors? *New England Journal of Medicine,* 362: 1066–9.

I found it harder to know what the following article was about without looking at its summary (which was more helpful).

Frank, MA (1981) Social indicators and health-for-all. *Social Science and Medicine. Part C: Medical Economics,* 15 (4): 219–23.

Abstract

The abstract is a precise summary of the whole report. It previews the contents of your report so that readers can judge whether it is worth their while reading the whole report. It includes a statement of the aim or objective of the investigation, a brief description of the method used and the main results, and the conclusions or implications of the results. The abstract should normally be a single paragraph between 100 and 200 words. Many design their abstract around IMRAD.

Writing abstracts is an art well worth cultivating. Your entire dissertation is captured in this section. It is absolutely your work and does not include any references. When people have to choose whether or not to select your work for presentation at a meeting, or to look up your paper online or in the library, it is only the abstract that they will look at. The trick is to be absolutely sure of your research question and to be ruthlessly honest about exactly what your results show. Keeping focused in this way easily keeps you within your word limit and makes the abstract a punchy summary of relevant work rather than a description of research people read with indifference. Read a few abstracts now and see which ones appeal to you – you'll see how easy it is to take or leave a paper based on this.

You might try writing abstracts of what you are reading both as a way to take meaningful notes and to check how well you've understood the point of the article (don't read the abstract until after you've tried writing one) or book. Activity 8.3 allows you to test this out.

ACTIVITY 8.3

Try writing an abstract for a journal article you've been told to read. If it comes with an abstract already, resist the temptation to read it first! You could then check your version against the original.

While abstracts for articles are usually about 150 words long, abstracts for dissertations are generally about 300 words long. The following case study shows how an abstract succinctly states what the much longer work is about.

Case study: An example of an abstract for a report on norovirus

Relevant background information is first given.

Worldwide, noroviruses are the major cause of acute viral gastroenteritis and reported incidence has increased in recent years, particularly associated with an outbreak strain in 2002. Although usually mild and self-limiting it is associated with mortality in developing countries and the immuno-suppressed and is highly transmissible, having a low infectious dose and being transmitted via the faecal–oral route.

This includes the rationale for the research.

Norovirus particularly affects hospitals, as they provide an ideal environment for rapid transmission and patients often experience more severe and prolonged symptoms than others. Hospital outbreaks result in ward closures and have associated costs to the health services and individuals affected. National guidelines were published in the United Kingdom in 2000, but there has been no evaluation of their evidence-base or their implementation in practice. It is possible that the increase in incidence has affected the extent to which hospitals are able to implement the guidelines.

Methods (evaluation through a literature review systematically undertaken, data collection, sampling and outcome measure stated)

A ... literature review was undertaken to identify the strength of evidence underpinning interventions to control outbreaks of norovirus in hospital. Fifteen NHS acute Trusts in South West England participated in a telephone survey using a semi-structured questionnaire to measure the extent to which their outbreak control policies are evidence-based.

Results

The results found that the national guidelines were evidence-based but did not score highly against an appraisal instrument, reflecting the difficulty in researching the effectiveness of infection control interventions, other than those which can be investigated in laboratory conditions. There is little research to demonstrate the effectiveness of those interventions in clinical settings. Hospital practice was largely based on current guidelines, but there was some discrepancy and variations in practice between the hospitals; for example, duration of ward closures.

Discussion

The study highlights the need for further research on effectiveness and suggests initiatives to improve practice and public health outcomes.

(McCulloch, 2007)

Introduction

As with essays, the introduction has a distinct function. It provides a rationale for the study and gives a clear indication of the argument to be developed. The introduction starts by giving the broad context within which your research fits, supporting points with reference to relevant literature. Explain the research paradigm, context and justification for the research (Chapters 1 and 4). Here you should also review the literature and provide a critical analysis of previous work (Chapters 2 and 3). A statement of your specific hypothesis or research question(s) is the usual way to end an introduction. This statement of the hypothesis should logically follow on from your literature review. It may be useful to make an explicit link between the variables you are manipulating or measuring in your study and previous research. For an example, see the introduction of **www.ncbi.nlm.nih.gov/pmc/articles/PMC2933355**

Methods

This chapter/section describes the methods of your investigation with enough detail that someone else could repeat it (see Chapters 4–6). Explain why the approach was chosen. Topics covered here should include: study design, study population, procedure for sampling and sampling frame used, inclusion and exclusion criteria, data collection methods, baseline and follow-up procedures (for longitudinal studies), data analysis and ethical approval. See the methods section of **www.ncbi.nlm.nih. gov/pmc/articles/PMC2933355**

Results

You describe your results to provide the reader with a factual account of your findings. Draw attention to specific trends or data that you think are important (in particular any disconfirming events). Use figures and tables to give a visual picture that is easy to understand (see Chapter 6). Your aim is to make your results comprehensible for your readers.

Where you have statistical results put descriptive statistics first (means and standard deviations) followed by the results of any inferential (analytic) statistical tests you performed. If relevant, indicate any transformations to the data you report. Only excerpts (descriptive statistics or illustrative highlights of lengthy qualitative data) should be included in the results section, and only those analyses that develop your argument should be included. Note that any results that challenge or refute your argument must be included.

When you describe a particular result, make sure you refer to its corresponding table or figure (diagram) in brackets after you have mentioned the results. The figures (diagrams) should be inserted into the text as soon as possible after you mention them. The lengthy results section in **www.ncbi.nlm.nih.gov/pmc/articles/ PMC2933355/** reports qualitative data and uses a table to give a timeline of events.

Discussion

Your fundamental aims for this chapter/section are to explain your results and to explore the significance of your findings. Thus you will:

- interpret and explain your results;
- examine whether and how the questions raised in the introduction section have been answered;
- show how your results relate to the literature;
- discuss the theoretical significance of your results;
- suggest any new research questions or areas for future research arising from your results.

The discussion is also where any reservations you have about the research should be signposted. Statistically significant results require discussion of their implications in the light of the research question. Chapter 7 covered this process in more detail.

References (or bibliography)

Citations are shortened references to the literature given in the body of text itself, and are minimal, for example, see World Health Organization (WHO, 2004) citation in the extract below. The full bibliographic details are then given in the reference section at the end. Be consistent in the referencing system you adopt. The Harvard system (author surname and date in the text) makes it easier to keep track of citations when editing. It provides a safety net for spelling of names: if the text citation differs from the reference then you can double-check. The Vancouver style (consecutive numbers linked to bibliographic details in the references section) is manageable for articles in scientific journals. If you store your references in an electronic reference manager (e.g. EndNote) then the program allows you to choose which reference style is required throughout the text and in the references section at the end.

Completeness and consistency of the references are important details to check. For instance, don't write John Black (2010) and then Coles, E (1991) in the next reference. And please help the reader by including the issue number as well as the volume number. A reference section called 'references' should only include materials that are cited in the text.

You may have read more widely than the articles you found useful for your argument. Sometimes you want to show how much reading you've done, particularly if very few references end up being used. Then it is useful to call this section a bibliography. A bibliography is a list of references relevant to the subject matter of a publication recommended for further reading; these include references not cited in the text. *The references within a bibliography should be presented alphabetically, according to the names of the authors. A bibliography may be subdivided into sections by subject, in which case items should be presented alphabetically within each section* (WHO, 2004, p5).

Appendices

Relevant appendices can include items such as copies of an interview schedule, forms for consent and letters giving permission for doing the research. Give each separate category of item its own title and number (see the hypertext appendices in **www. ncbi.nlm.nih.gov/pmc/articles/PMC2933355**).

Posters and presenting at conferences

It is important to start attending scientific meetings. You'll see your team in a different light, socialise with them in a different setting, become comfortable with networking, and gain confidence about showcasing your work. The number of conferences is growing every year in different places, close by or overseas. You can find out when they are from the medical education units in your medical school, postgraduate centre, the departments you work in, the library, online advertisements and, of course, from your peers and teachers. Send off an abstract, ask for help and advice and you may be pleasantly surprised to find how easily your work is accepted.

Scientific meetings enable scientists to present their new work to their colleagues to get feedback at an early stage of their research. They are an integral part of the scientific process. Do take advantage of attending meetings, seminars and conferences. You'll meet people and find out what is going on and you'll gain an understanding of 'how things work'.

Creating a poster is an excellent start to attending conferences. You don't really have to talk to anyone if you really can't face it and you have a gentle introduction to conferences where you can hear other people speak and see other people's work without really being seen yourself. Don't forget the poster has already been accepted as an abstract so you really can't lose, no matter how you design the poster. There are usually competitions for the best one but it isn't usual to have to stand with your poster and present it to anyone verbally.

When you design the poster, keep your research question central and make it obvious. Make sure your results address the question directly and have conclusions that are clear to someone glancing at the poster from ten paces away. The temptation is to have too much information, lots of graphs, tables and images. This will just look like splashes of colour and the message will be lost if you can't confine yourself to the essentials that convey your message most effectively.

You can type and design the poster on a PowerPoint slide and e-mail it for printing in the medical school, hospital or copy shop in the high street. If you are presenting as part of a group or organisation, there may be an organisational template to use. The conference website always has instructions on the dimensions and specifications and you can always e-mail or telephone the organisers with queries. Don't ask for the deluxe printed version when you know you're not going to display it again and again in the department or over the mantelpiece. It won't be long before you build up a collection. Be meticulous about typographical errors (typos). Seeing them on a piece of paper that represents you forever in large scale is hugely disconcerting.

Presenting a poster, or even making a presentation, is an excellent way of getting to know other people and to display your findings. People will approach speakers/contributors to find out more about their study, and you'll feel more a part of things. Tips on poster preparation can be found on **www2.le.ac.uk/offices/careers/pgrd/resources/designing-poster/poster**. Effective posters are legible with a clear message, and sited at a height that's easy to read. The people you want to impress may have rickety knees, so don't pitch important points too low down.

Don't be afraid of presentations. When you send an abstract to a conference they may accept your abstract either as a poster or as an oral presentation. An oral presentation is brilliant news. As a medical student you really can't go wrong. The entire audience is behind you, willing you on and incredibly impressed that you undertook a piece of work, saw it through and have now come to present it. They know how hard you've worked and are entirely on your side.

What you must do, and extremely experienced people seem to forget, is look up on the conference website exactly how long the presentation is to be. People always forget or misread the instructions, preparing a 15-minute talk when it's supposed to be ten minutes long with five minutes for questions. Rushing through the last few slides ruins an otherwise memorable presentation.

When you prepare your slides, remember not to have too many words on each slide, to have as few slides as possible altogether (typically one slide per minute of presentation or less) and to check for typos again and again. Typos shouldn't be discovered for the first time in the middle of the presentation as this is a source of embarrassment for most presenters.

Customise the title slide with your name, your team, the institution, the conference title or logo and the date. Presentations where words flash or fly across the slides usually fail to impress. Keep the special effects to a minimum, the colours conservative and check that the colour scheme allows the word to stand out from the background.

Credit references you use, e.g. on the slide below, and look at other people's slides to see how they have done this. Lots of styles are equally correct and effective (Figure 8.2).

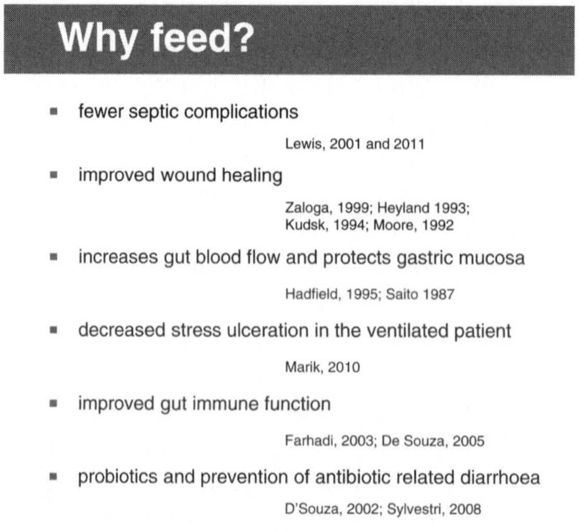

Figure 8.2 Referencing examples.

If the presentation is more than five minutes or comprises different parts, make your second slide a contents slide. Always have take-home messages at the end and finish with a slide of references listed in the Vancouver style.

Really know your slides and practise the presentation again and again so that it is polished and seamless. You should not need to look at the slides to know what's next. Never read your slides. Look at your audience, relax and talk. Keep to time!

Novices often seem to think that presentations should entertain when actually they should explain. Use graphs to show the shape of the data, and from that shape discern meaningful patterns, such as trends and exceptions. Make sure that the most important parts of the message stand out above all else. When you are deciding which type of graph to use for your situation, the decision tree on the weblink below can help you. The key questions to consider are whether the data are time-sequenced and how many data series you want to show. By selecting the appropriate graph type, you can help make the message clearer to the audience. **www.thinkoutsidetheslide. com/articles/using_graphs_and_tables.htm** has free resources about using PowerPoint. There are many sources to help with the effective use of PowerPoint (Pugsley, 2010).

Do not worry about the questions at the end. You are not defending your results, you are presenting them, emphasising their significance, explaining problems that arose during the research and clarifying points to the audience that they may not have heard the first time or are genuinely interested in. It is a compliment to be asked a question: at least they were interested and want to know more. It is universally acknowledged by doctors and researchers that presenting to your own department is infinitely harder than at a conference. If asked a question you cannot answer, admit it, don't flounder. If it would take time to explain properly, ask the person to see you at the coffee break (that's what such breaks are for).

The use of blogs and wikis

James Heilman (Clinical Assistant Professor at the University of Saskatchewan), in a posting to the listserv **HIFA2015@dgroups.org** (accessed through **www. hifa2015.org/**) on 10 August 2011, explained that Wikipedia does have many controls in place. The first line of defence:

> is a series of computer scripts that automatically reverts obvious vandalism / spam. There are than [then] lists of recent changes to the text that are gone over by a group of volunteers to check their accuracy. Users who are interested in a topic also keep articles on their 'watch list' to be notified if changes are made. Articles that are subject to high levels of disruptive edits can have the editing of them restricted to established registered users.
>
> Really controversial subjects may only be editable but [by] administrators of the site (for English there are about 900 admins). And specific images have at times been locked into place to deal with their frequent removal.
>
> Single users or internet addresses which are disruptive on an ongoing basis may have their editing privileges removed. While Wikipedia has a very open editorial policy

it is not a free for all (even though it may sometimes seem like this). Wikipedia has a peer review process.

Articles are rated based on quality and good articles receive a review by at least a single other editor while featured articles receive a second round of reviews by multiple other editors. Thus we are able to generate some exceedingly high quality content. While one might not get the accolades that one receives by publishing in a journal what one writes on Wikipedia matters as this is where much of the world including professionals get their health information (Wikipedia get 150–200 million page views for its 23,000 English medical articles a month and exists in approximately 250 other languages).

Increasingly medical schools are opening facilities for students to develop their own blogs and wikis. This collaborative form of learning does not replace coffee shop conversations but potentially extends them. In posting to and using such media it is most important to enact what you have learned about ethics/professionalism and confidentiality. Using these to disseminate your research makes possible international collaboration with like-minded people. Use the dialogue to sharpen your ideas and the networking to expand your horizon.

Technological developments create new opportunities for working collaboratively in order to improve health outcomes. An outbreak of a new strain of *Escherichia coli* in July 2011 in Germany affected more than 4,000 people. The use of **crowd-sourcing**, open-source genomic analysis and an open approach to the release of data rapidly identified the causative pathogen and facilitated control (Rohde *et al.*, 2011).

Writing for publication in peer-reviewed journals

There are many reasons for you as a medical student to try to publish. Here we discuss the competitive advantage publication may give you when it comes to applying for jobs, opportunities in medical journalism for those interested in this for a short period or a future career, and finally, writing to give you a voice independent of the rest of the college faculty. Certainly, opportunities to write are increasing as more journals seek student editors and try to cater for students rather than junior doctors, and more student blogs develop into student publications. Firstly, we discuss in some detail why and how to publish clinical material.

Competition is a way of life for most medical students and trainees. All medical schools have percentiles or a ratings system that remind students of where they are in comparison with their colleagues and by the time students think of intercalating a further degree or sitting prize exams they have started to look for ways to distinguish themselves. Publishing papers is one way in which to achieve this. By the end of medical school, application forms for the Foundation years score publications and presentations and competing for training posts is equally hard, if not harder. Although scores can be totalled up from a myriad of achievements, publishing research, audits or case reports is an excellent way of demonstrating academic achievement and a lasting evidence of your interest in aspects of medicine you have encountered in your training (Activity 8.4).

ACTIVITY 8.4

Do the points just mentioned resonate with you? Find out what opportunities exist for you to show what you are capable of in your programme.

It is unlikely that you will be able to publish audit research when in medical school. Unless your medical school curriculum facilitates achieving a full audit cycle (Chapter 9), it is difficult to find a finite audit project that can be undertaken in the short period of time that you are attached to a team as a medical student and then prepare and submit a manuscript while you are with the same clinical team. Audits are, therefore, much easier to undertake after qualification when life on the wards really begins for you and all Foundation doctors will carry out a clinical audit. Although increasingly medical students are encouraged to consider their role as change agents, it is likely that examining a clinical process and trying to improve it will happen after you have become a doctor. However the fresh eyes of novices can see potential for improvement that escapes those set in their ways. It's to be hoped you'll find opportunities to share these ideas with clinical staff, and that they are generous enough to acknowledge your contribution.

The first experience of publication for some students may well be writing a case report. Writing up a memorable case with your team is a valuable learning experience. It is the opportunity to investigate further about a case, search the medical literature, find and compare clinical guidelines, ask probing questions about the pros and cons of management decisions and, most of all, explain your point of view in the medical literature.

As evidence-based medicine goes, case reports are level 5 evidence (below clinical trials and case series) but case reports do have their place. We learn from our discussion of cases we manage every day. It helps to discuss unusual presentations, complex symptoms, ethical or practical challenges, near-misses, pitfalls and how complications may present and are dealt with. The debate is an educational one and case reports are an ideal educational resource for real case-based discussion. A common perception is that only rare or novel cases are worthy of publication. In fact, we learn far more from common cases that present in an unusual way or common management pathways that meet an impasse or result in an unexpected outcome.

Tips for writing up a case report

Find a clinical case with valuable educational lessons for junior doctors or medical students. The patient may be someone you meet as a student on your clinical attachments, or, indeed, a patient you looked after on a medical student elective. After gaining the patient's consent take any clinical pictures you need to illustrate your points and then type up the case using the following structure.

- Summary – Try to project the lessons of value and points of interest so that these are immediately apparent to someone else reading your case. You may choose to write this section last, as your report takes shape, but this will be what captures the attention of your audience.

- Background – This is essential information that sets the scene and explains why certain symptoms or complications may have arisen during the course of illness.

- Case presentation – For most of us this is frequently the easiest section to begin writing. This is an outline of everything that happened to the patient from the time of presentation to discharge. This is ideal for you to write as you are most likely to have completed most of the case note entries yourself and merely need to consult your notes. Be sure to include all relevant results and write these in full using internationally recognised units and explaining abbreviations, for example: 'The patient was hypotensive with a blood pressure of 130/80mmHg and had developed neutropenic sepsis with a WCC, white blood cell count, of 2.1×10^9/l'.

- Investigations – This is where radiological images illustrate your results and good pictures are extremely effective.

- Differential diagnosis – Rather than listing these, it is crucial to demonstrate how differential diagnoses were formed and diagnoses excluded as the patient was worked up. Clinical reasoning is fascinating as an entity in itself, but case reports are a brilliant opportunity to demonstrate how diagnoses are teased out through clinical problem-solving. This is where case reports really earn their place among other medical literature.

- Treatment – The best case reports present the case, investigations, diagnosis and treatment as an honest and reasoned process where management decisions are explained clearly. Clinical judgements and treatment plans, therefore, make immediate sense, especially to a doctor of a different specialty.

- Outcome and follow-up – These give the clearest idea of the progress of a case. All too often this is neglected as inpatient teams may be disconnected from outpatient care. This information is crucial, however, and tracking a patient's progress after discharge is, of course, excellent practice for the inpatient team.

- Discussion – There is no need for the discussion to be a summary of all the literature about a particular clinical problem. Focus on points that make the case notable and where lessons can be learned. This may be a mechanism of injury, a pitfall in the interpretation of investigations, the suitability of appropriate clinical guidelines, necessary departures from these guidelines or their adaptation in a particular scenario, the management of challenging complications – there are innumerable possibilities.

- Learning points and take-home messages – These are essentially your final conclusions and serve to crystallise your thoughts on exactly why you think this case is of value and what we can learn. You may find this very effective in focusing your thoughts when you begin typing the case report.

- The patient's perspective – This may be a most enriching contribution. We urge you to involve patients in the process from the beginning, as doing so is likely to result in a well-rounded account and the process of obtaining consent for images and publication is rendered more meaningful.

Submitting medical images with a brief clinical summary is also an effective way of becoming published, so do look out for spectacular images that provide opportunities for learning.

Writing for a journal is different from writing for academic purposes. What you write has to be slanted so that the topic is appealing to the audience reading the journal, and also complies with the way in which the journal presents itself to its readers. This is described in the following section.

Write with an audience/journal in mind

When Cochrane was asked to give the Rock Carling lecture (later published as *Effectiveness and Efficiency*: Cochrane, 1972) he began by thinking about his potential audience (non-medical intellectuals and medical students). Focusing on the core idea of improving the NHS through use of randomised controlled trials he decided *to keep the book short and simple, with a few jokes to assist its palatability* (Cochrane and Blythe, 1989, p237). It is time well spent to read 'instructions to authors' when you have identified journals that are likely to accept your article (because they tend to publish similar types of research). Make sure you comply with their instructions. Really strategic writers will look up the 'impact factor' of journals and send/apply to the highest-rated one first. You should wait for the first to reject you (being pessimistic!) before sending it to another. Do not give up if the manuscript is rejected but ask for feedback, learn from it and send it to the next journal in your list.

House style of journals

House style is the preferred spelling, punctuation, terminology and formatting to be used for the various information products published by an organisation. Within WHO headquarters, British rather than American spelling is normally used. The general rule is to follow the spelling listed in the latest edition of the *Concise Oxford Dictionary* (the few exceptions are flagged in the WHO *Style Guide*: WHO, 2004). The WHO *Style Guide* is a large volume of instructions for all authors writing WHO reports, journals or technical documents. All journals (and many organisations too) also have their own house styles which can be found under 'instructions to authors'. It's a way of standardising writing so that any article has the flavour favoured by the journal. Readers 'know what to expect'.

Two example instructions are:

1   *All abbreviations should be defined and spelt out the first time they are used, unless likely to be familiar to readers. A few abbreviations, such as e.g., i.e., etc., are so widely used that the complete words are almost never given. The World Health Organization (WHO) was established on 7 April 1948;*

2 *It is not acceptable to refer simply to Laos, Libya, Syria or Tanzania. These countries must be referred to as 'the Lao People's Democratic Republic', 'the Libyan Arab Jamahiriya', 'the Syrian Arab Republic' and 'the United Republic of Tanzania', respectively.*

(WHO, 2004, pp3 and 14)

As a matter of fact, reading that statement on how to express names of countries correctly is rather telling of the WHO's apolitical status, as Activity 8.5 shows.

ACTIVITY 8.5

Take this point further by using a search engine to find 'WHO style guide' (WHO/IMD/PUB/04.1). Read pages 10–12, 14–17, 31–2 and 85–93 to find out how the WHO perceives the geographical world.

Make your argument clear and relevant

Writing well, honing your skills in getting your point across with appropriate grammar and vocabulary is a skill. You acquire this through publishing more than through any written assignment in medical school. It really matters that you can make your assertions clearly and explain how you came to your conclusions. The peer review process is rigorous, usually with more than one reviewer going through the manuscript and they are candid in their comments. The process of responding to their criticism and shaping the manuscript into a paper of which you can be proud is a great exercise in writing. You are likely to find that your writing in general is improved and you are better able to see the wood from the trees in patients' past medical histories. This is of great value when you come to sit your final examinations and have to present information succinctly, with the most salient points clearly leading to a well-argued list of differential diagnoses.

Issues relating to co-authorship

Students and trainees who undertake research are encouraged to work with their teams or supervisors on research papers. You may or may not be the first author on a publication but a research paper will serve you well when it comes to applying for Foundation or subsequent training if you are first author. Indeed, students with prior degrees who apply to study medicine are encouraged to publish their prior research.

It is a courteous convention that PhD students invite their supervisor to co-author their first publication in a peer-reviewed journal. People also may co-author research publications with colleagues/other team members. Both are acknowledgements that research is a joint enterprise in which people collaborate and their contribution should be acknowledged. The benefits of jointly writing material stem from the intellectual stimulation, the ability to play to individuals' strengths and potential efficiency. Responsibility is shared, and novices learn and benefit from the expert authors' know-how and networks. Journals now require the contributions of authors to be identified to ensure there are no 'free-riders'. An early decision needs to be agreed as to the principle for deciding which name goes first. With citation indexes affecting promotion prospects, being first or second author is prized. Academic communities vary as to how they sequence authors after the first author, especially for large teams, so check conventions. If someone has given good advice and ideas or reviewed your paper helpfully, then you should mention this in an 'acknowledgments' paragraph. Funding sources and conflicts of interest need to be stated.

Co-authors need to share assumptions about what is important. If they cannot agree then the partnership is doomed, at least for that publication. Many scientists will withdraw their name on a paper rather than be associated with an analysis or conclusions they feel are unsupported by the data. That is acting with academic integrity.

Copyright

Copyright law protects the author of a work from others copying it without written permission. While the author of a set of lectures or seminar papers has the right to turn them into an article or book, a student who heard the lectures and took verbatim notes has no right to so do, and if given permission must cite the source author. The copyright holder has the right to refuse permission (and would certainly refuse if he or she disapproved of the use to which an item was put) and to charge for use. You must remember the possibility of copyright infringement whenever you include another person's words, figures, graphs or photographs in any work you publish. This is a legal matter so try to secure written permission beforehand. Simply attributing the source (so as to avoid plagiarism) is not sufficient; copyright law is enforceable and its requirements differ in different countries.

Creative commons

Increasingly researchers are building sites that give free access to their work provided it is properly acknowledged. They are known as 'open source' sites. It is not always free without requesting permission from the owner so it's important to read what is needed in order to use materials.

Moral rights

In addition to the right of licensors to request removal of their name from the work when used in a derivative or collective they don't like, copyright laws in most jurisdictions around the world (with the notable exception of the USA, except in very limited circumstances) grant creators 'moral rights' which may provide some redress if a derivative work represents a 'derogatory treatment' of the licensor's work.

Chapter summary

- It is important to respect the rights of creators of knowledge to be recognised.

- The aim of disseminating the findings of any investigation is to build good practice.

- Opportunities to disseminate your work in a variety of ways should be seized.

GOING FURTHER

Becker, H (2007) *Writing for Social Scientists: How to start and finish your thesis, book or article*. Chicago, IL: University of Chicago Press.

Join an online community of writing practice (open source): **www.oercommons. org/courses/writing-commons/view**

Global Health Education Consortium (with links to tips on writing): **globalhealth education.org/resources/Pages/default.aspx**

World Health Organization (2004) *Style Guide*. **thailand.digitaljournals. org/community/download/6**
There is good sound advice here for writing in general and furthermore you gain an insight into the WHO as an organisation.

Taylor and Francis: *Publishing in Academic Journals*. **www.vimeo.com/21687973**
The process of submitting a paper to a journal and understanding the peer review process are both explained in this video podcast. You will also find out how to choose the best journal for your paper and how to prepare the 'perfect' manuscript and learn ways to improve your chances of publication, including the top ten reasons for rejection.

Instead of intercalating a BSc/MSc you may decide to spend a year in medical publishing or medical journalism. There are a number of opportunities available if this interests you. One example is the Clegg scholarship at the *British Medical Journal*. This is an opportunity to gain real experience of the world of medical journalism for a few weeks, and if this is something you would like to pursue, becoming a student editor is an excellent idea. The *student BMJ* has a medical student editor. The post is for a year, after which you would resume clinical medicine, having formed contacts in an environment where you might wish to pursue a career eventually. There are similar posts available with other medical journals, for example, the *Journal of the American Medical Association* has the *Medical Student JAMA* which, like the *student BMJ*, also invites the full range of articles from doctors, researchers and students, including scientific and creative writing. **jama.ama-assn.org/site/misc/aboutmedicalstudentjama.xhtml**

There is an ever-increasing list of medical student publications, quite apart from local college gazettes, with further opportunities for publication experience, such as the *International Journal of Medical Students* (**www.ijms.info/index.php/ijms**). These provide opportunities to write widely on issues affecting medical students and do not require the submission of clinical material. They give students a voice and are a platform for students to discuss their views independently of doctors or a wider faculty.

chapter 9

Audit

Dawn Lau and Ann K. Allen

Achieving your medical degree

This chapter will help you to begin to meet the following requirements of *Tomorrow's Doctors* (General Medical Council, 2009).

Outcomes 3 – The doctor as a professional

20. The graduate will be able to behave according to ethical and legal principles. The graduate will be able to:

   (b) Demonstrate awareness of the clinical responsibilities and role of the doctor, making the care of the patient the first concern.

21. Reflect, learn and teach others.

   (c) Continually and systematically reflect on practice and, whenever necessary, translate that reflection into action, using improvement techniques and audit appropriately – for example, by critically appraising the prescribing of others.
   (f) Function effectively as a mentor and teacher including contributing to the appraisal, assessment and review of colleagues, giving effective feedback, and taking advantage of opportunities to develop these skills.

The chapter will also enable you to meet the UK Foundation Curriculum (Academy of Medical Royal Colleges, 2012) requirements for engaging in and understanding research, audit and evaluation.

It will also introduce you to the following professional standards as set out in the core curriculum for *Good Medical Practice*, as published by the General Medical Council (2006):

• Paragraphs 12–19

Chapter overview

After reading this chapter you will be able to:

• explain what a clinical audit is and what it can achieve;
• explain how clinical audit fits into the context of the changing NHS and clinical

governance;
- understand your own role in clinical audit;
- describe how to design and carry out a clinical audit;
- use a range of sources (including the internet) to search for standards and evidence when designing an audit;
- identify relevant ethical concerns (including patient consent) and practical issues

Introduction

Clinical audit involves the review of healthcare-related activity data against predefined **standards** or **guidelines**. Its primary purpose is to improve quality by promoting adherence to standards. It is a cyclical process of assessing current services against set standards, taking actions to bring practice in line with the standards and reviewing whether these actions have had the desired effect. Combined with feedback to, and education of, clinicians and medical students, clinical audit is a tool that enables clinicians (and the teams in which they work) to improve the care they provide to patients, and thus to build clinical **effectiveness**.

This chapter will first look at what clinical audit is, explore why it is important and how it is implemented, using case studies to help you understand how this essential healthcare activity contributes to improving quality in the delivery of healthcare services. You may be invited to participate in a clinical audit as a medical student and you certainly will as a Foundation doctor, so it is important that you understand the 'bigger picture' it serves.

This chapter also introduces key organisations and their place in the audit network and process, including:

- the National Institute for Health and Clinical Excellence (NICE);

- the Healthcare Quality Improvement Partnership (HQIP);

- National Clinical Audit and Patient Outcomes Programme (NCAPOP);

- various specialist societies, such as the British Thoracic Society (BTS).

The stages of the clinical audit cycle will be explained so you will feel confident you know how to conduct and appraise one.

What is clinical audit?

The term 'clinical audit', first coined in 2002, spells out an approach to quality improvement based on clinical data collected by health professionals, so as to improve their patients' quality of care. It is a tool for health professionals to improve clinical care, rather than a management or regulatory tool.

Clinical audit has many differently expressed definitions. One internationally recognised definition comes from 'Principles of Best Practice in Clinical Audit':

> *Clinical audit is a quality improvement process that seeks to improve patient care and outcomes through systematic review of care against explicit criteria and the implementation of change. Aspects of the structures, processes and outcomes of care are selected and systematically evaluated against explicit criteria. Where indicated, changes are implemented at an individual team, or service level and further monitoring is used to confirm improvement in healthcare delivery.*
>
> (Clinical Governance Support Team NHS, 2005, p3)

Read the case study below.

Case study: Concern for improving clinical care is not new

The concerns underpinning clinical audit are not new: what was new from the 1990s was a concerted application throughout the NHS of assessing practice against prescribed standards.

You're probably familiar with the story of Florence Nightingale and her reform of clinical conditions in the military hospitals in Scutari in Turkey following the discovery that French soldiers fighting in the Crimean War received much better medical care than the British soldiers. Use of detailed reports in what was effectively an audit that she carried out to persuade key stakeholders (politicians, administrators and generals) of the need for change was backed up by a judicious mix of negotiation, persuasion and political influence to bring such change about. Her social position was as helpful as her clinical acumen in this respect.

Over half a century later, Abraham Flexner, a research scholar at the Carnegie Foundation for the Advancement of Teaching, undertook an assessment of medical education in the USA and Canada. He carefully documented the many problems which contributed to doctors being poorly trained. His 1910 report prompted major reforms in medical education to entail scientific and properly supported clinical training. Again, this was an early form of clinical audit.

Concern in Britain with maternal mortality led to a series of periodic enquiries or audits from 1932 onwards. Better guidelines for patient management as a result of this audit process improved the care provided, which lowered maternal mortality rates. From the outset it was guaranteed that such reports would be treated with absolute confidentiality and they would not be used for disciplinary purposes (Crombie *et al.*, 1993).

Evidence-based medicine

Prior to evidence-based medicine (EBM) (discussed in Chapter 2), clinical decisions rested on custom and anecdotal practice (Illich, 1974). Now, EBM underpins all clinical audit. National Framework Standards and national guidelines are based as far as possible on the best available evidence that has been rigorously scrutinised by NICE. Other important sources are specialist society guidelines and Scottish Intercollegiate Guidelines Network (SIGN). The clinical audit standards are referenced back to their source and an explanation of this link is usually provided. Where there is no evidence base, consensus standards are developed and agreed through an appropriate consensus methodology (for example, using the **Delphi technique**) among experts in that particular field.

Now complete Activity 9.1.

ACTIVITY 9.1

Choose a clinical topic of interest, then select a clinical practice within that specialty which is accepted and routine, such as the use of antibiotic prophylaxis against infective endocarditis for invasive procedures. Is there much evidence behind this practice or treatment? If you want to find out what research evidence suggests the best care option, it is worth looking at two websites that summarise a lot of research:

- The Cochrane Collaboration for health care: **www.cochrane.org/index.htm**
- The Campbell Collaboration for social care (including education and crime and justice): **www.campbellcollaboration.org/index.shtml**

An example of a clinical intervention which came under the spotlight several years ago was the use of antibiotic prophylaxis against infective endocarditis for invasive procedures. Until 2008, it was routine practice to offer antibiotics as a preventive measure to patients at risk of infective endocarditis who were undergoing interventional procedures, including dental and other endoscopic interventions. There has been insufficient evidence to prove this practice to be effective and there is no clear association between episodes of infective endocarditis and interventional procedures. This was therefore reflected in NICE guidance (NICE, 2008) which recommended that antibiotic prophylaxis should not be routinely prescribed for certain defined invasive procedures, recognising that any benefits from prophylaxis needed to be weighed against the risks of adverse effects for the patient and of antibiotic resistance developing.

Investigations that are not clinical audit

Routine monitoring is not the same as clinical audit. As explored in other chapters, investigations, or data collection and analysis, may be initiated for many different purposes. Analysis and interpretation transform data into information. Both are influenced by the purpose. Routine monitoring and audit serve different purposes. Routine monitoring records information that is useful for managers, such as:

- patient admissions' data, for instance, record information that a manager needs to know about length of stay/throughput of patients;

- staff absence due to sickness is relevant for monitoring staffing levels/the need to employ locums/payroll accounting.

Sometimes these records may be used by others with different purposes but it would be a happy accident if the data recorded for administrative tasks were exactly fit for a different purpose.

Data collection is only one component of clinical audit, which must also include comparison against explicit audit criteria, reflection of the data gathered and a plan for improving care.

There are also other forms of data collection which do not constitute clinical audit (as discussed elsewhere): research, surveys, patient registry, patient-reported outcome measures, patient satisfaction surveys and service evaluations.

What's the evidence?

In practice, clinical audit is not applied consistently. This illustrates the conceptual confusion about purpose that prompted us to write the book you are reading.

[T]here is a diversity of opinion in what constitutes clinical audit at the NHS front line of service provision, with considerable overlap between clinical audit, the components of service evaluation and the requirements of organisational development; and its relationship to quality improvement not always evident. These factors influence the degree to which its effectiveness can be evaluated.

In its formal, agreed, best practice form, clinical audit is designed to measure compliance with standards of proven clinical practice and record the required and documented changes in clinical practice that arise from improvements that are introduced. Many audits identified in the CiREM review however do not get to re-audit stage; still less of them to repeated cycles of audit.

(HQIP/Cambridge Institute for Research, Education and Management (CiREM), 2011, pp11 and 49)

The differences between the various quality improvement methodologies are discussed in more detail in Chapter 1, Table 1.3, which will help you compare and contrast and remain clear about the appropriateness of each methodology.

What clinical audit can achieve

So why is clinical audit important? As you have seen from the previous section, it is imperative that healthcare should not be a static process but that we continue to seek ways to improve it for the ultimate benefit of patients. The NHS has been evolving in recent years to become more focused on the quality agenda. In 2008, Lord Darzi published the White Paper *High Quality Care for All*, which calls for quality to be the core element of service delivery and clinical practice (Secretary of State for Health, 2008). It also defines three broad components of quality:

1. patient safety;
2. clinical effectiveness (application of best knowledge from research; experience and patient preferences to achieve optimum processes and outcomes of patient care);
3. the patient experience.

Clinical audit provides an integral component of delivering the quality improvement agenda of the Darzi report.

Clinical audit may promote best practice, which should confer benefits to patients both in their experience of care and health outcomes. It provides evidence of where clinical services are effective and efficient, as well as giving opportunities for learning and education.

Improving care through change

The audit cycle must include reflection on the data gathered and establishing a plan of action to improve care (we will look at the audit cycle in more detail next). There may then be further rounds of data gathering and reflection to ensure standards are improving. However, a problem with demonstrating the effectiveness of clinical audit arises from the fact that audits are seldom repeated (HQIP/CiREM, 2011). Unless you look to see what has happened (reaudit), you cannot know what's changed. The following case study succinctly illustrates the use of audit to improve the care pathway of patients who are admitted with acute asthma.

Case study: Clinical audit associated with improvement to patient care

Clinical audit of the acute management of asthma in a busy district hospital in England revealed both good practice points as well as areas for improvement. This audit was conducted as part of the BTS national audit programme which allows all hospitals within the UK to participate, thus enabling each hospital to compare its audit results with the national average and BTS standards. The time interval for prospective data collection was two months.

Initial measurement against standards

The majority of adult patients admitted with acute asthma had an admission peak expiratory flow (PEF) measurement in order to compare it with their usual best. All of the patients with oxygen saturations in the low 90s% had an arterial blood gas done. All the patients were discharged with a prescription of oral steroids.

Aspects of care which needed improvement included subsequent PEF monitoring of inpatients, documentation that inhaler technique and compliance had been checked and respiratory outpatient follow-up within four weeks.

Change implemented

- Consideration of more asthma specialist nurses to be involved with the management of all asthma patients admitted.
- Continued training of junior staff within their teaching rota and induction day to encourage good documentation and ensure these patients are educated before discharge, with help of the asthma nurses.
- A renewed commitment by the respiratory department to prioritise the follow-up appointments of these patients to ensure they are reviewed within four weeks of discharge.

Patient benefit

A reaudit after a year is being done to chart the progress of the implementation plans to ensure patients are shown to be benefitting, thus aiming to complete the audit cycle.

The case study shows how, through audit, areas for concern can be identified. Because professionals (and the organisations they work for) are likely to be concerned about the consequences of reporting failure, it is important to develop a blame-free culture when conducting a clinical audit so it is more likely that such information will be shared. Well-conducted clinical audit enables *the quality of care to be reviewed objectively, within an approach which is supportive, developmental and focused on improvement* (HQIP, 2009). It is not conducted to apportion blame – rather the aim is to review current practice against ideal standards of care, so as to identify ways in which care can be improved.

As well as improving patient care, audit can improve communication between clinicians, managers, patients and organisations. The case study below illustrates this.

> **Case study: Improvement in communication as a result of an audit**
>
> *As a result of one of the audits taking place on the learning disability ward new software has been purchased and adapted to allow for the development of easy read care plans (pictorial representation of the care plan). This has promoted inclusion and accessibility as it allows those with learning difficulties to be involved (despite difficulties) with agreeing, updating and reviewing their care plans.*
>
> (HQIP/CiREM, 2011, p38)

It's important to be aware that *interprofessional and organisational dynamics such as leadership, hierarchies, clinical attitudes to new learning, and so on . . . influence implementation* (HQIP/CiREM, 2011, p5). As well as improving the quality of clinical care and ensuring the improved safety of care provision, audits satisfy the policy requirement for accountability and financial imperatives to deliver care efficiently and provide value for money.

Accountability

Healthcare workers are made accountable through asking them to follow guidelines and protocols about what to do in particular situations. Conducting a clinical audit encourages staff accountability for performance both individually and as a team.

People are held accountable for their actions in different ways and at different levels. These include explicit statements about their responsibilities, official mechanisms for examining performance (e.g. in the appraisal and revalidation of doctors, participation in audit activity must be demonstrated), as well as processes for investigating when things go wrong (e.g. with clinical incident reporting). For doctors, the responsibility of improving the quality of care is enshrined as a professional requirement within the General Medical Council guidance *Good Medical Practice* (2006), and is assessed through clinical audit.

Keeping records is part of what makes employees accountable for their actions. But a risk of creating many formal accountability structures is that clinicians can spend time and energy writing up their activities at the cost of providing the best-quality care through building relationships with patients.

Accountability of health institutions can be further facilitated when hospitals publish the reports of their completed audits and publicise them. This means interested service users could read them and:

- have access to good-quality information to help them make choices about their care;

- through knowing what has happened in the past, know what to expect in the future.

Is this last point just a wishful hope? Activity 9.2 should give you some ideas. Bear in mind that ultimately it is the patient who has the greatest interest in the best clinical practice.

ACTIVITY 9.2

Find out which of your local hospitals publish any reports on quality and safety. Are they available to the public or only within health trusts/boards? To help you, navigate the website of the health institution to which you are currently attached and see if you can find the right documents. How easy or difficult is this process?

Darzi's White Paper emphasized the need to:

- measure quality (need to measure and understand what we do in order to work out how to improve);

- publish quality performance (*making data on how well we are doing widely available to staff, patients and the public will help us understand variation and best practice . . . and focus on improvement* (Secretary of State for Health, 2008, p48).

Training and education

An increasing part of medical training and medical practice goes beyond clinical knowledge and skills: medical leadership training, quality improvement and associated change management techniques are essential tools for ensuring high-quality and improving care. Participating in clinical audit is an opportune way to learn these skills, and goes beyond formal medical or specialist training to become part of continuing professional development. You may also learn presentation skills, negotiation and understanding of change within complex healthcare systems.

The development of clinical governance and clinical audit in the NHS

To understand the role of clinical audit it is useful to know something about its background. Since its establishment in 1948, the UK NHS has been concerned with the quality of the healthcare it provides. In 1980, *Inequalities in Health* (known as the Black Report after its chairman Sir Douglas Black) was published by the British government (Department of Health and Social Security, 1980); this report revealed that, although overall health had improved since the introduction of the welfare state, widespread health inequalities associated with social class existed. This led to recognising the need for audit to compare and reduce inequalities.

Other research studies also contributed to the growth of audit. For example, Cochrane's seminal book *Effectiveness and Efficiency* (1972) led to the use of randomised controlled trials to create evidence for the effectiveness of therapeutic practice (thus providing an evidence base for the audit of practice). Avedis Don-abedian, the authority for quality measurement in healthcare (Bashshur, 2003; Don-abedian, 1978), suggested a framework for the evaluation of the structure, process and outcomes of medical care so as to safeguard and enhance the quality of care. This helped create a context whereby publicly provided healthcare became expected to be efficient and grounded in evidence. The creation of NICE in the 1990s to appraise evidence and cost-effectiveness formed the evidence base on which many clinical guidelines and standards are based.

Clinical governance

Clinical audit is part of a wider process of quality monitoring known as **clinical governance**. Clinical governance is defined as:

> *A framework through which NHS organisations are accountable for continuously improving the quality of their services and safeguarding high standards of care by creating an environment in which excellence in clinical care will flourish.*
>
> (Department of Health, 1989, p33)

Concern for governance has its origins in the commercial sector, following a number of high-profile misdemeanours in the private sector. Clinical governance mirrors this accountability and responsibilities of corporate governance in the area of health service quality. By April 1991 audit was expected to be implemented in every hospital by all consultants. The 1997 White Paper *The New NHS: Modern, dependable* (Department of Health, 1997) required NHS trusts to report in what was known as a **performance framework** on the following six areas:

1. health improvement;
2. fair access to services;
3. effective delivery of appropriate healthcare;
4. efficiency;
5. patient/carer experience;
6. the health outcomes of NHS care.

Chief executives and medical directors in the NHS became directly accountable for the quality of the services provided by their organisations. Structures and processes for effective clinical governance were put in place by 1999. Quality monitoring and improvement thus became a core component of routine trust/health board management rather than an 'optional extra' only undertaken in the wake of a public scandal or by enthusiasts. Clinical governance was given further impetus by the Bristol Royal Infirmary Inquiry (2001) costing £14 million, as is shown from the case study below.

Case study: Bristol Royal Infirmary Inquiry

It is 27 October 1998. A preliminary hearing of the public inquiry into the management of care of children who received complex heart surgery between 1984–1995 at the Bristol Royal Infirmary is being held, chaired by Sir Ian Kennedy. This has been triggered by alarms raised that the mortality and morbidity rate of children undergoing open heart surgery had been higher than expected, and has separately led the General Medical Council (GMC), preceding the Inquiry, to hold a disciplinary case against two Consultant paediatric cardiac surgeons and the hospital manager. They have since been found guilty of serious professional misconduct: one surgeon and the hospital manager have consequently been struck off the GMC register, and the other banned from operating for three years.
(Department of Health, 2002)

The Bristol Royal Infirmary Inquiry lasted for nearly three years, and took evidence, both verbal and written, of over 500 witnesses, including about 200 parents. The inquiry also received 900,000 pages of documents, including the medical records of over 1,800 children. It found that the systems for paediatric cardiac surgery (PCS) in Bristol, and the NHS in general, were flawed, resulting in one-third of all the children who underwent open-heart surgery receiving inadequate care. More children died than might have been expected in a typical PCS unit: from 1991 to 1995 between 30 and 35 more children under a year old died after open-heart surgery in the Bristol Unit than might be expected had the unit been typical of other PCS units in England at the time.

The public inquiry found some of the culture and flaws which sadly contributed: the lack of appropriate facilities and specialist-trained staff, including lack of a full-time paediatric cardiac surgeon; presence of a 'club culture' manifest as an imbalance of power, with too much control in the hands of a few individuals; a system of hospital care which was poorly organised and beset with uncertainty as to how to get things done, such that when concerns were raised, it took years for them to be taken seriously. It also highlighted a lack of agreed means of assessing the quality of care. There were no standards for evaluating performance. There was confusion throughout the NHS as to who was responsible for monitoring the quality of care.

The inquiry produced nearly 200 recommendations which broadly encompassed a number of themes: prioritisation of very sick children, safety, competence of healthcare professionals, organisation, standards of care, openness and monitoring of performance.
(*Source:* www.bristol-inquiry.org.uk/final_report/the_report.pdf)

Clinical audit is the principal method used to monitor clinical quality. Monitoring the quality, effectiveness and outcomes of care is both a means of encouraging clinicians to improve their practice continuously, and also a mechanism to build awareness of the developing evidence base that informs clinical guidelines and standards. Other clinical governance structures operating within the NHS include:

- critical incident reporting and review;

- patient surveys and complaint management;

- peer review processes such as morbidity and mortality meetings and appraisals.

The organisation of audit today: national and local audit

To ensure that the potential of clinical audit is maximised, the Department of Health launched a renewed initiative in 2008 which saw the formation of HQIP, which commissions and performance-manages national clinical audits funded by the Department of Health. Through NCAPOP, HQIP oversees national projects that provide trusts with a common format for data gathering and support and develop the contributions of these local departments. The projects analyse the data centrally and feed back comparative findings to help participants identify necessary improvements for patients. Most of these projects involve services in England and Wales; some also include services from Scotland and Northern Ireland. The National Advisory Group on Clinical Audit and Enquiries (known as National Clinical Audit Advisory Group before 2012) advises the Department of Health on audit priorities.

All NHS trusts are expected to participate in the national audit programme. Participation is usually spearheaded by individual healthcare professionals who evaluate aspects of care that they themselves have selected as being important to the local service. Such audits are known as local clinical audits. HQIP works to foster these 'bottom-up' local clinical audits and supports networking between trusts that are auditing the same topic. You can find examples of local case studies at **www.hqip. org.uk/case-studies**. Students and junior doctors are encouraged to participate in consultant-determined local audits as part of their professional education. There are also regional or multisite audits which involve not just one local service, but all services at a regional level, and these can provide useful opportunities for **benchmarking** and cooperation.

We have looked at the standard-setting organisations; at the other end of the spectrum, standards are monitored for quality assurance by bodies such as the Care Quality Commission, Monitor (which regulates foundation NHS trusts) and the National Patient Safety Agency. At the local level, trusts and health boards have a statutory responsibility to define, report on and ensure explicit qualities of care.

Who is involved in clinical audit?

Consultants may take the lead in deciding to undertake a clinical audit but Foundation doctors particularly and medical students are encouraged to participate. Service users should be part of the clinical audit process and the clinical team should be multidisciplinary. Involving service users in service delivery at every stage, from planning through implementation, to review and monitoring is a means of ensuring care provision is patient-centred, and this is why it is recommended that they are involved in the audit process.

Case study: Medical student involvement in improving patient care

It is quite possible that you as a medical student or Foundation doctor may see opportunities for improving patient care yourself. This is taken from a year 3 medical student blog:

> When the baby came out he was very blue, not breathing and when I checked his heart rate it was beating … below 60bpm (guidelines say that if a newborn's heart is 60 beats per a minute then you should initiate chest compressions). So AJ and I and a midwife initiated resuscitation, suctioning (the baby had a lot of secretions in his lungs) and rubbing/lightly pinching the baby to try and stimulate the baby into taking a breath. When it came to cardiopulmonary resuscitation I was doing the chest compression and … AJ took over the bagging and the midwife … came back over to check everything was going ok. It was better when it was just AJ and me doing the resuscitation because the midwife was instructing us to do the wrong CPR ratios – we had looked up the current guidelines for newborn resuscitations following the caesarean the other day when the other medical students had ended up doing CPR on that baby … I'm definitely going to try and find a way to educate staff about CPR now.
>
> (www.newmediamedicine.com/forum/weblogs/ 54085-half-doctor-hits-wards-2.html#post769594)

It is the clinical professionals who are responsible for collecting and checking data as they have the specialist skills: analysis may be done by clinical audit staff, usually located within a centralised department. If you are asked to undertake a clinical audit as a part of your studies you should find out where the clinical audit team is located and take the initiative to contact them. Apart from being able to advise you about your proposed investigation, they will be able to suggest clinical audit projects that fit with wider programme planning. They can also help with the retrieval of case notes and data support. That will mean your investigation will not distract from local commitments and that your results are likely to be relevant.

Activity 9.3 shows what can be achieved by those with the will, whatever their motivation for undertaking an audit.

ACTIVITY 9.3

Listen to the four-minute podcast: 'You'll win nothing with kids'. You will find this on the Clinical Audit Support Centre podcast link: **www.clinicalauditsupport.com/ podcast/podcast.html**.

This podcast highlights how every member of the healthcare team can make a difference, including junior members.

How you may be involved in clinical audit

As a medical student it is likely that you will participate in data collection and analysis for a clinical audit even if your curriculum is not set up so that you can complete a full cycle. As was shown earlier, the effectiveness of clinical audit is handicapped by the lack of published reports, the variable quality of what is reported, and the fact that clinical audit cycles are seldom repeated. A better approach is to involve medical students or junior doctors in contributing to different stages of the audit cycle:

- identifying standards for an audit;
- carrying out the data collection, reflection and developing an action plan;
- working with senior colleagues to help drive change arising from the action plan;
- carrying out a reaudit so as to take this cycle forward.

If you ask questions about why recommendations made in earlier reports were not implemented you may learn about organisational and other constraints, and so better prepare yourself for future practice. Also, as you saw earlier with the student (who wrote she was going to *educate staff about CPR now*), it is vital you speak up if you think a mistake is being made. This may lead to a clinical audit being undertaken.

The clinical audit cycle

The clinical audit process may be viewed as a cycle (or spiral heading upwards), as shown in Figure 9.1.

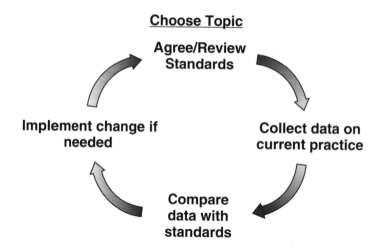

Figure 9.1 The audit cycle.

The process of audit involves a series of steps.

1. Select your audit topic.

2. Determine the aims and objectives of the audit.

3. Identify standards of best practice and establish the audit criteria.

4. Collect data.

5. Analyse data against the previously identified standards and reflect on findings.

6. Feed back the audit results – getting the message across.

7. Discuss possible changes and implement them.

8. Allow time for changes to become established before reauditing to record progress.

Each of these steps will be explained in turn.

Select your audit topic

The choice of topic for a clinical audit is usually based on a clinical concern at local level or maybe an audit that has been made mandatory at national level. It may also be triggered by adverse events, patient complaints or user reviews or new research evidence.

What makes an appropriate topic to audit? Topics should:

- be of interest and importance to clinicians – this might be because the subject is high-risk or high-profile;

- be of relevance to the department and the way it delivers care, as well as to the trust management – this may include a service or intervention which may be high-volume or high-cost;

- have availability of established and authoritative standards and measurable criteria;
- lead to service improvements that are achievable within your resources;
- involve a clearly defined population to be audited.

Consult with your clinical colleagues and with the Audit Department of the trust about this. This should result in high interest and maximum staff and patient involvement. Where other sectors are involved in patient care it is important to ensure they participate from the outset. You need such 'buy-in' if changes are to be implemented successfully.

Case study: The problem of risk of venous thromboembolism (VTE) in acutely ill medical patients

VTE is a major health problem both in the community and within the hospital. It may lead to both mortality and morbidity, including post-thrombotic venous insufficiency and ulceration, affecting quality of life and healthcare costs.

Most cases of VTE (deep-vein thrombosis and pulmonary embolism) occur in medical patients. In 2005, The House of Commons Health Committee produced a report on 'The prevention of VTE in hospitalised patients' which estimated that 25,000 people in the UK die from preventable hospital-acquired VTE every year. Although there are safe, efficacious and cost-effective prophylactic methods, they are not as widely administered as they should be and there was no systematic approach to preventing VTE-related deaths. In response, the Chief Medical Officer set up an independent expert working group that reported back in April 2007 with recommendations for VTE prophylaxis in higher-risk medical patients in the form of low-molecular-weight heparin (LMWH) subcutaneous injections and/or antiembolism stockings.

At one of the NHS trusts, an audit in December 2005 showed that only 30% of acute medical patients at risk of VTE and without contraindications received appropriate VTE prophylaxis. More locally within the trust, there has not been an audit of VTE prophylaxis use within the Chest Unit, where a significant number of patients would be expected to have severe respiratory disease as well as important comorbidities.

We shall use this example to work through the audit cycle.

ACTIVITY 9.4

From the case study, what is the particular topic that you think is important to audit? What are your reasons?

Having selected the topic you now identify the precise areas that will be the focus of your study.

Determine the aims and objectives of the audit

The next step is to clarify the aims and objectives of your audit.

- Aim: Why are you doing this project? What are you trying to achieve?
- Objective: Define your aim more precisely – what aspects are you seeking to improve?

Don't try to achieve too much. Your project should be achievable within a reasonable timeframe and with the resources you have. Failure to complete the audit is disheartening for everyone involved and a waste of resources, including time.

ACTIVITY 9.5

You've decided that doing a clinical audit on VTE prophylaxis on your medical ward is appropriate. What would be your aims and objectives for your clinical audit?

If you were really undertaking this clinical audit, this is when you would compare your ideas with the Chest Unit team.

Case study: Establishing the clinical audit aims

The team on the Chest Unit agreed that auditing on the topic of VTE prophylaxis on their ward is clinically important. The aims of the clinical audit were:

- to assess documentation of risk assessment of patients admitted to Chest Ward
- to ascertain incidence of VTE prophylaxis use within the Chest Unit, measured against the 'gold standard' of _____ guidelines.
- to document LMWH use in case notes.

The team contacted and engaged with the Audit Team within the trust and registered the audit so that it became part of the trust's audit programme.

The next step in the audit cycle is to find and agree standards of care to which you aspire.

Identify standards of best practice and establish the audit criteria

It will be impossible to identify areas for change and improvement unless the standards are expressly stated and audited against. This involves:

- selecting the audit criteria (elements of care or activity, which can be measured);
- setting your desired level of performance or target (the level you are aiming for, such as the number or percentage of patients you would wish to meet or achieve that criterion).

The terms 'standard', 'protocol', 'guideline', 'guidelines', 'guidance' and 'pathway' are all used interchangeably in different contexts (Ilott et al., 2006).

Donabedian (1966) stated that in order to measure quality, there are three dimensions to consider:

1. the structure of care – how care is delivered (facilities available, numbers and skills of staff);
2. the process of care – what care was delivered;
3. the outcome of care – the result (recovery, for instance).

Structures are relatively easy to measure as they do not usually require the identification of patients' case notes. An example is assessing the number of trusts that have a full complement of staff trained to deliver a service. However, even if an audit shows organisational structures are in place, this may not imply better care for the patient.

Process measures assume that if people receive care that is gold-standard, then outcomes should be good. Assessing process of care will require retrieving data from case notes. This is time-consuming and poor record-keeping can affect interpretation. Despite this, it is easier to obtain than outcome data in complex chronic conditions. An example of process-type criteria would be whether a patient got the care/tests/treatment recommended by evidence-based practice.

Outcome measures relate to:

- measures of access to care (waiting times, referral pathways);
- results from care (blood pressure reduction in response to therapy);
- direct measures such as death, complication or survival.

Whilst outcomes are the ideal measure for assessing quality they can be difficult to assess. Survival is a particularly difficult outcome measure as it requires both case-mix adjustment (that is, adjustment of variations in confounding variables between populations under study) and often lengthy follow-up. It is important to ensure that like is compared with like to get a fair picture. Data need to be 'risk-adjusted' to standardise for factors such as age, severity, case mix and concurrent illnesses. Outcome measures are likely to differ between clinical specialties and procedures. For example, death rates might be a good measure of outcome after cardiac surgery, but for hip joint replacements a better measure might be how long the new hip lasts or postoperative infection.

ACTIVITY 9.6

Find out where and what the clinical standards are for VTE prophylaxis in medical patients admitted to hospital. Read them, and note down the standards you want to measure the care against.

You would then want to identify suitable criteria so you can measure performance of clinical management against the standards.

Case study: Selecting criteria

NICE issued clinical guidelines (CG92) in 2010: 'Venous thromboembolism: reducing the risk', which were mirrored by the local trust guidelines which could be accessed within the trust intranet. The medical team set out the gold standards based on the NICE guidelines, paying particular attention to the guidelines' 'key priorities for implementation'.

- All patients admitted to the Chest Unit should have documented risk assessment for VTE, including any documented risk of bleeding.
- Pharmacological VTE prophylaxis (in this case dalteparin) should be offered to general medical patients assessed to be at increased risk of VTE.

Criticisms of the use of standards

Some practitioners claim that following guidelines or protocols can deskill the workforce in aspects of analytical reasoning, especially when guidelines are followed unquestioningly. Some complain they are being introduced for the wrong reasons:

- pressure from insurers;
- the hospital 'covering its back';
- managers being able to blame individuals rather than acknowledge failures in the system.

Some also worry that protocols limit flexibility and that care becomes less individualised. The quality of the research on which the protocols and guidelines are based may be met with scepticism – no piece of research will tell you the best way to proceed with every single person. Professional judgement and freedom are considered to be limited by protocols, particularly when commissioning care packages (for example, recommending the use of a specific drug for a condition) may give rise to later questioning about doctors' decisions in relation to the care of a specific patient (when another drug considered better for that particular patient was used).

Collect data

The next part of your audit is collection of the data to measure level of performance. There are many sources of established standards which can be transformed easily into audit pro formas (a data collection tool which comprises specific criteria to measure reality) and these should be used in the development of clinical audit studies. Rather than trying to design one yourself, it is more useful to apply an existing tool first and then adapt it later if you need to. Specialist society, National Service Frameworks or NICE guidance is helpful for locating data capture tools which may either be paper- or electronic-based.

Data collection may be either retrospective (looking back in time) or prospective (following over real time). A prospective clinical audit collecting accurate real-time data reflects current rather than historical practice and may yield better-quality data. Retrospective audit increases the possibility of identifying all patients meeting the inclusion criteria provided that there is appropriate coding to capture these cases. However, tracking down case notes or incomplete documentation can cause problems. It's usually more practical to do a retrospective audit, especially if there is a time restraint for producing results, or if there are limited resources and staff to follow up on cases. Focusing on process measures rather than outcome is also more practical. Activity 9.7, on collecting the data to capture criteria-relevant performance for the VTE audit, applies these ideas.

ACTIVITY 9.7

Design a simple pro forma. How will you decide on numbers of cases to audit or timeframe for patient 'capture'? How will case identification be possible? Will it be retrospective or prospective – how will you decide?

A one-page pro forma with simple tick boxes included:

- baseline patient characteristics;
- the list of risk factors which would trigger consideration for VTE prophylaxis;
- the contraindications for VTE prophylaxis;

- if a note had been made in the admission clerking if the patient should have dalteparin;

- whether dalteparin was charted/given;

- if prophylactic dalteparin was not given, were there any contraindications?

Case study: Measuring level of performance

Drawing on NICE guidelines, the medical team created a data collection tool, as detailed above. They conducted a retrospective audit for one month as the throughput of patients on the Chest Unit was high. The case notes were identified using electronic admission data and retrieved with the help of the Audit Team.

The sample chosen for audit should be small enough to allow for rapid data acquisition but large enough to be representative. In some audits the sample will be time-driven (for example, one to three months) and in others it will be numerical (for example, the numbers of case notes to be retrieved). National audit studies have suggested that approximately 40 sets of case notes are required to provide a view of care in a healthcare setting. If the data acquisition time is too long, interest will be lost and data completeness may suffer. Don't forget that, particularly in regard to time-related audits, the seasons can have a dramatic effect on such samples. In both primary care and the acute sector, process audit often shows deterioration in the winter and this should be taken into account by your audit design.

Clinical audits do not need to undergo the lengthy and rigorous processes needed to gain formal ethical approval. Soliciting consent for the retrospective analysis of case notes is also impractical and it is assumed that permission is implied because the purpose is to review them in order to improve the standard of care and data are anonymised.

Analyse data against the previously identified standards and reflect on findings

After you have collected your data, you then need to analyse the data against the standards that you identified earlier. Data analysis can vary from straightforward numbers, percentages and averages to more complex statistics. As a general rule, keep this as simple as possible so that everyone in the team can understand how results have been obtained. Analysis should be easily understood by patients and managers if the audit is to be useful for planning constructive changes.

Clinical audit is directly related to improving services against a standard that has already been set by asking the following five questions:

1. Is what ought to be happening actually happening?

2. Does current practice meet required standards?

3. Does current practice follow published guidelines?

4. Are clinicians applying the knowledge that has been gained through research?

5. Is current evidence being applied in a given situation?

How this is done is shown in the case study below.

Case study: Analyse the results against the explicit criteria

Here is a snapshot of what the medical team found:

- Dalteparin documented:
  - 18/51 (35%).
- Dalteparin given:
  - 30 given dalteparin:
    - 5 treatment dose;
    - 27 prophylactic dose.
  - 13 had contraindications not to have dalteparin:
    - 1 recent spinal surgery with concern re: haemothorax;
    - 5 on warfarin;
    - 6 mobilising;
    - 1 ?GI bleed.
  - 33/51 (65%) patients satisfied criteria for prophylactic dalteparin.
  - 8/33 patients not given dalteparin with no contraindication/reason documented = 24%, i.e. 76% of patients who should be on VTE prophylaxis are receiving this.

The team reflected on the findings.

- The majority of patients in the Chest Unit are at risk of VTE: 65% of these were eligible for VTE prophylaxis.
- 76% of eligible patients were receiving dalteparin – much higher compared to the 2005 hospital audit result of 30%, reflecting increasing awareness.
- There was poor documentation in patient notes re dalteparin use (35%); none had checklist forms completed/entered into notes.

The final stage in your audit cycle is to feed back the reaudit results to all key stakeholders, which include trust management, clinical team and audit department.

Feed back the audit results – getting the message across

There are a number of important avenues to get your message across and the presentation of findings should be readily understandable and include:

- the background of why you chose the topic;

- the method (patient eligibility criteria, gold standards, compliance expected with the standard – is 100% reasonable?);

- your results and analysis and comparison with previous rounds of audit if appropriate;

- a plan of action to address the weakness identified in the service or care.

Case study: Presenting the clinical audit

The team presented their audit results at the trust's audit Annual General Meeting where a good attendance of clinicians ensured the topic was highlighted more widely. The audit report was also sent to the clinical lead consultant of the Chest Unit for ward dissemination among staff.

Other potential local avenues include trust newsletters or bulletins, clinical meetings, feeding into trust governance systems through management and using the trust intranet. Wider dissemination can facilitate **benchmarking** with other hospitals by feeding into specialist society audit systems or clinical audit networks at regional or national level.

The next stage in the audit cycle is to examine possible changes that are needed as a result of your analysis, and then to implement them.

Discuss possible changes and implement them

This is where clinical audit can become more political. It is very important to respect people's sensitivities and constraints so as to propose a workable intervention (Bohmer, 2010). You will remember the purpose of clinical audit is to improve performance: this may involve people needing to be trained or more closely supervised; it may involve additional costs; it may involve people feeling threatened (Carthey et al., 2011). While whistle-blowing has become somewhat acceptable, revealing all on a blog or to the Sunday papers is not the most effective way of getting things done differently. Remember how diplomatically Florence Nightingale convinced the sceptical military doctors that her nurses had a useful role to play.

Having identified problems or deficiencies in structures and processes or poor outcomes, clinical audit must develop an action plan to improve the structures or process of care. The action plan is a list of practical steps to be taken within a timeframe. Members of staff responsible for specific actions are identified. This should lead to an improvement in outcome.

In many instances, process improvement alone may have to be used as a surrogate measure for outcome improvement, particularly in those areas where the projected outcome improvements are either small or of long duration (for example, improvements in thrombolysis times should improve mortality from myocardial infarction but it is impractical to wait for confirmation). In surgical specialties outcomes may be more obvious (the provision and appropriate use of high-dependency facilities will reduce cardiovascular, renal and respiratory complications and thus the risk of death).

However, even with true outcome audit, the investigator will still need to know what parts of the process may have contributed to poor outcomes. This will come from either published research or local expert knowledge. The use of core people actively suggesting how things could be improved will tap into this local expertise.

Case study continued

The medical team came up with a number of recommendations.

To improve the appropriate use of prophylactic dalteparin through:

Guideline dissemination:

- induction of new doctors both at trust level and within the department;
- easy availability of risk assessment checklist by including it as part of the patient admission clerking pro forma;
- inclusion of VTE prophylaxis measures in the trust drug chart.

Continuing education:

- a teaching session as part of junior doctor weekly teaching timetable;
- during ward rounds with specialist registrar or consultant.

Clinical audit – to close the audit loop

The VTE Implementation Working Group, with input from stakeholders and key partners, had developed a VTE risk assessment for use in all hospitals (Appendix 3: **www.dh.gov.uk/en/Publicationsandstatistics/Publications/PublicationsPolicyAndGuidance/DH_088215**)

- – Discussion regarding trust-wide adoption of Department of Health checklist to ensure standardisation?

The next step is to develop an action plan of how things might be improved practically, who will do what and within what timeframe. An example of an action plan is illustrated within the *Template clinical audit report* on the HQIP website: **www.hqip.org.uk/template-clinical-audit-report**

Allow time for changes to become established before reauditing to record progress

The last stage in your audit cycle is to do another audit, after you have allowed enough time for changes to become established. It is estimated that 90 per cent of audits with an action plan need be reaudited. Hopefully that reaudit would then demonstrate improvements. If this is sustained, some form of monitoring should replace a full audit which could be reactivated if performance deteriorates. This will retain enthusiasm in the audit process and allow a more innovative approach to patient care. Reaudit involves:

- collecting a second set of data;

- analysing the reaudit data.

The HQIP/CiREM (2011) review of evidence of the impact of clinical audits demonstrated three fundamental components of effective clinical audit:

(1) There have been repeated cycles of audit.

(2) It is likely that audit was carried out in a methodical manner.

(3) Change in clinical practice and resultant effect have been recorded and analysed.

Let all discuss whether practice has improved: if people see benefit and feel ownership, it is more probable another audit will be welcomed. There is a need for training and encouragement to follow best practice and to start to measure outcomes from the outset.

Chapter summary

- Clinical audit is:

    o first and foremost a professional and clinical tool, not a management or regulatory tool;
    o to evaluate local clinical practice against guidelines about best practice;
    o to improve patient care and outcomes;
    o to ensure clinical practice is based on the best available evidence.

- The importance of clinical audit lies in:

    o improving quality of care;
    o accountability and General Medical Council requirement;
    o training and education.

- Clinical audit is a part of the wider concern with clinical governance and the expectation that clinical staff will continuously update their knowledge, understanding and skills.

- The structures and organisations associated with clinical audit include NICE, specialist societies and the HQIP, among others.

- An outline of 'how to do a clinical audit' and complete the clinical audit cycle was given.

GOING FURTHER

www.clinicalauditsupport.com/podcast/podcast.html
Clinical Audit Support Centre released free podcasts in a range of formats, including news updates, blogs, interviews and panel discussions to inform about key developments in the world of clinical audit and quality assurance. These podcasts can be listened to via the iTunes store. Started in 2007, they give insight into the issues in the practice of clinical audit, though the most recent was posted last in early 2011.

HQIP *Literature on the Effectiveness of Clinical Audit.* **www.hqip.org.**
uk/literature-on-the-effectiveness-of-clinical-audit
These are reviews on the effectiveness of clinical audit, both within the UK and internationally.

www.nice.org.uk
NICE provides guidance, sets quality standards and manages a national database to improve people's health and prevent and treat ill health.

www.evidence.nhs.uk/frequently-asked-questions
Evidence NHS gives access to a collection of guidelines for the NHS. It is based on the guidelines produced by NICE and other national agencies.

www.uhbristol.nhs.uk/for-clinicians/clinicalaudit/how-to-guides
The University of Bristol has developed a series of easy-to-understand-and-apply articles about clinical audit for students and clinicians new to audit.

chapter 10

Doing Health Service Evaluation and Quality Improvement

Ann K. Allen and Dawn Lau

Achieving your medical degree

This chapter will help you to begin to meet the following requirements of *Tomorrow's Doctors* (General Medical Council, 2009).

Outcomes 1 – The doctor as a scholar and a scientist

12. Apply scientific method and approaches to medical research.

   (c) Apply findings from the literature to answer questions raised by specific clinical problems.

Outcomes 2 – The doctor as a practitioner

19. Use information effectively in a medical context.

   (b) Make effective use of computers and other information systems, including storing and retrieving information.
   (d) Access information sources and use the information in relation to patient care, health promotion, giving advice and information to patients, and research and education.

Outcomes 3 – The doctor as a professional

20. The graduate will be able to behave according to ethical and legal principles. The graduate will be able to:

   (b) Demonstrate awareness of the clinical responsibilities and role of the doctor, making the care of the patient the first concern. Recognise the principles of patient-centred care, including self-care, and deal with patients' healthcare needs in consultation with them and, where appropriate, their relatives and carers.

21. Reflect, learn and teach others.

   (a) Acquire, assess, apply and integrate new knowledge, learn to adapt to changing circumstances and ensure that patients receive the highest level of professional care.

The chapter will also enable you to meet the UK Foundation Curriculum (Academy of Medical Royal Colleges, 2012) requirements for engaging in and understanding research, audit and evaluation.

Chapter overview

After reading this chapter, you should be able to:

- explain what evaluation is;
- discuss the purposes of a health service evaluation;
- describe the essential components and approaches of a health service evaluation;
- describe the basics of designing and carrying out health service evaluation;
- describe the basics of quality improvement.
- explain why safety matters and what is involved to promote it in healthcare.

Introduction

Professionalism in medicine means maintaining high standards of practice and constantly striving to improve the quality of clinical care a patient receives. As a doctor you will sometimes be hampered from achieving these goals by circumstances that relate to the working environment. This is where evaluating health services can help. Audit, which was discussed in the previous chapter, evaluates clinical practice and service delivery against expected standards (associated with protocols, guidelines and National Service Frameworks, for instance). Health service evaluation takes stock of what is happening in order to see what could be done better or even sometimes if a service should continue to be offered. Both audit and health service evaluation contribute to the medicosocial movement that has become known as quality improvement. See Table 1.3 in Chapter 1 for a summary of the differences between these approaches. This chapter starts by building your understanding of evaluation and its purposes, then the essential components and approaches to health service evaluation are described. The different steps to do one are described. Following this the basics of quality improvement and how patient safety can be promoted are outlined.

What is evaluation?

A medical student has been turned down by a leading aid agency for an elective attachment – they say they need qualified doctors with experience and training in safety and security.

Upset by this, he decides to see whether only doctors are of use to aid agencies rather than students. Is he alone in wanting to do an elective with an aid agency? Are other students interested? If there are enough medical students really interested in working with aid agencies, will he be able to show his research to an aid agency and convince them that they should set up opportunities for student electives? This student is undertaking research for the purpose of evaluation. He hopes to find evidence that will convince the agency that it is worth their while to change their policy and consider medical students' applications. He believes that what medical students lack in experience as doctors they can make up for by being dutiful, helpful and resourceful in other ways that may benefit the agencies. In other words he wants to evaluate what those students who go in fact do and whether they are helpful.

The purpose of evaluation is to see what changes need to be made (and sometimes, if something should continue). Think back to the last time you considered the need to make a change. Before you decided on a particular course of action, you would have had to analyse that situation. You may have considered:

- What problem prompted the need for change?

- How should you approach resolving the problem?

To help you decide what needed changing, you probably identified the positives you wanted to keep. That left the things that might need changing. Additionally, you would consider available options, weighing up how well each met your particular need and comparing advantages and disadvantages of each to inform your decision-making. Unlike in an audit there is no predefined 'gold standard'. To facilitate any change, you have to work through this sort of process, which is known as **evaluation**. You probably did this kind of evaluating when you were applying to medical school. Which university to choose – the one nearest home or the one your friends from school were going to? You might even have wondered if medicine was the right career choice for you, and weighed it against other options such as registering for one of the sciences or even taking the risk of forging a musical career with your band.

A broad definition of evaluation is the assessment and determination of the quality or value of something (Robson, 2000). Evaluation is applied in all aspects of society: from the personal, social groups and the workplace, to government and government organisations (e.g. how cost-effective is it to run the Forensic Science Service?), as well as international organisations (e.g. how effective was the World Health Organization's response to the H1N1 pandemic?). Sometimes evaluation is termed a 'review'. Reviews are usually carried out in order to improve or change systems or organisations. Other broader formal activities which involve evaluation include public inquiries, for example the Bristol Royal Infirmary Inquiry (Chapter 9).

Implicit decision-making processes work for most day-to-day choices people make about their lives. In areas such as education and healthcare, evaluation needs to rely on a series of steps that are rigorous and systematic, because any decisions made have a much wider influence. The process of quality improvement in health services (whether of a programme, a service, an innovation or an intervention) requires following the cycle shown in Figure 10.1.

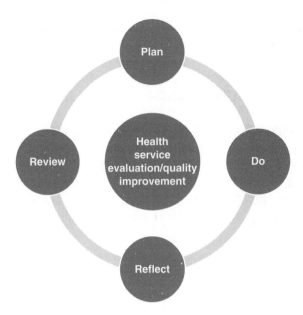

Figure 10.1 The cycle for health service evaluation/quality improvement.

The purposes of a health service evaluation

There are many reasons to evaluate. A positive reason is to improve a programme but there are also 'hidden' reasons, like finding a justification to close a service. Many employees find involvement in evaluation inescapable, and may lose sense of the greater purpose of why it's done beyond that of 'requirement' and bureaucracy. Reasons to conduct an evaluation may be broadly divided into two categories. The first is to look for areas for improvement, for example of a course, programme, teaching activity or clinical service. This is known as **formative evaluation**. The second is to assess and form a judgement of the value and merits of whatever one is evaluating, usually for decision-making and accountability purposes – this is known as **summative evaluation** (Robson, 2000). Examples of situations where summative evaluation is used include:

- comparison between 'competitors', for example league tables of universities;
- accountability to the public, for example, the General Medical Council's Quality Assurance of Basic Medical Education (QABME) programme ensures UK medical schools maintain standards, and involves regular monitoring and visits to medical schools;
- marketing purposes, for example student choice of a course;
- allocation of funds and resources.

(Davidson, 2005)

In reality, there is often a combination and overlap of intentions and reasons, albeit with differing degrees of emphasis. Activity 10.1 encourages you to think about how there may be a variety of intentions and reasons for an evaluation, particularly where different groups of people are involved.

ACTIVITY 10.1 A POSSIBLE EVALUATION

A big teaching hospital proposes to change the organisation of consultants' ward rounds from twice weekly to twice daily on the medical wards. This initiative was prompted by ongoing concerns relating to rising hospital costs, hospital-acquired infection and risks of thromboembolism because of excess average length of stay (ALoS). It was believed that the cause of these delayed transfers of care was a lack of senior decision-making that could be redressed by twice-daily consultant-led ward rounds.

- Who are the people or organisations who have an interest in this proposed change in practice? List them.
- Now putting yourself in their shoes, can you think of as many reasons as possible why this new arrangement should be evaluated? Do the reasons differ depending on the group of people?
- Keeping the list of your reasons in mind, formulate a variety of questions that you would like your evaluation to answer.

We shall be returning to your answers later in the chapter. Activity 10.1 was based on a real health service evaluation that you can read about for yourself.

Case study of a health service evaluation

Evidence from research in Liverpool showed how changing medical consultants' practice from twice-weekly to twice-daily ward rounds reduced the ALoS of patients by 50%, without an increase in either readmissions or mortality. It did not increase the working hours of the consultants nor other staff, and was cost-neutral (Ahmad et al. (2011) www.ingentaconnect.com/content/rcop/cm/2011/00000011/00 000006/art00005). We shall be using this example to illustrate the steps of carrying out a health service evaluation in a later section so you should download the article for future reference.

We now turn to how you might take part in a health service evaluation as a medical student.

How you may be involved in health service evaluation

You might get involved in such an activity for a student selected component, or it might form a senior clinical project for you. One way many medical students become involved is as stakeholders evaluating their clinical placements. Medical schools rely on the contribution made by NHS staff in teaching their students clinical skills and the tacit (not formally described) knowledge of how to behave professionally. So you may be asked to complete a questionnaire where there are items such as the following.

The learning outcomes identified in the Module Handbook were (for a particular hospital):

- very useful;

- useful;

- not very useful;

- not at all useful.

You would circle the answer you felt applied to you and then respond to a further question, which is 'Any comments?'

Responses such as:

- 'More specific learning points as to topics to learn would be very useful. The grid of "things to see" isn't very clear, especially for the histopathology/haematology section.'

- 'The tick box/experience gained system was not very useful. Also some procedures stated that we were only to observe, eg ABG which we should be competent in by the end of the block.'

These are helpful summative comments because they give details about how the learning experience can be improved, so they also perform formatively.

On the other hand, responses such as:

- 'A syllabus would be of more use for finals'.

- 'Not really possible to get all this done'.

- 'You use the all opportunities and situations you find yourself in to learn have a list read from is pretty useless.' (sic)

These comments, expressing dissatisfaction, leave the evaluator guessing how best to improve matters for future students. This last point may leave you wondering why people bother to evaluate if it's not going to benefit them. This is why – as will be explained later – formative evaluation takes place while there is still time to improve matters. However, as part of an ongoing professional responsibility to improve practice, students are required to give feedback even if it does not benefit them directly.

The next section reviews the essential elements of any kind of evaluation.

Essential components and approaches in evaluation

There are many dimensions to consider in any evaluation:

- **stakeholders** – persons or organisations with an interest (or stake) in something – in this case evaluation – or an interest in its success because they are involved in or are affected by it;

- reasons to evaluate;

- questions needing answers;

- do you measure outcomes (the results) or processes (activities)?

- formative versus summative purposes for evaluation;

- indicators (factors or variables that provide a simple and reliable means to measure achievement, to reflect changes connected to an intervention or to help assess performance).

These will be discussed in detail later.

Approaches to evaluation

Through the lens of evaluation, any service can be seen to be made up of facets, each (or all) of which can become the focus of an evaluation. The terms 'programme', 'service', 'change', 'intervention' and 'innovation' – whatever you may be involved in – are used interchangeably as we discuss evaluation principles. Evaluation can be categorised in different ways, as can be seen from the three approaches below. Robson's (2000) model is expressed diagrammatically in Figure 10.2.

1. Donabedian's (1966) distinction between structure, process and outcome (explained below) initiated the whole process of the evaluation of health services to improve the quality of clinical care. Robson's model modifies this to take account of economic concerns about needs and efficiency.

2. Robson (2000) classifies evaluation approaches based on needs, processes, outcomes and efficiency. The prospective elective student might look at what the agency needs (What are the routine organisational tasks that medical students could safely meet?); processes (Can the presence of a temporary volunteer be accommodated within the work schedule of a team of busy people?); outcomes (Can the student by clerking and checking equipment free up staff time so that they can heal patients?) and/or efficiency (Will the cost of supervising the medical student be outweighed by the benefits of increased numbers of patients treated?).

3. Another well-known evaluation model used to evaluate training courses looks at their effectiveness by measuring participants' reactions (satisfaction), learning (knowledge gained), behaviour (application of learning) and results/impact (Kirkpatrick and Kirkpatrick, 2006).

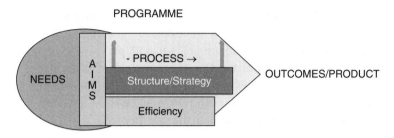

Figure 10.2 Types of evaluation.

The concepts referred to in Donabedian's and Robson's approaches are now explained before looking at the steps to take in doing a health service evaluation.

Evaluation of needs

For any new service, potential users of the intervention should be consulted as to their needs; this evaluation is also called a needs analysis. Other evaluations of needs are whether the users' needs are being met by the intervention (evaluation of outcomes), or whether what goes on when the intervention is in operation is regarded as satisfactory (evaluation of appropriateness).

Evaluation of structure

Structure refers to the conditions under which healthcare is provided. Examples of evaluations of structure include material resources evaluation (e.g. equipment, facilities); human resources evaluation (e.g. professional and support personnel); as well as evaluation of organisational aspects (e.g. medical staffing, methods of paying for care, presence of research and teaching functions).

Evaluation of processes

Evaluation of process relates to how a service is implemented. They are the activities needed to bring about a change in outcome. So whilst a vaccination programme aims to reduce the incidence of measles (outcome) it will not do so if children are not vaccinated, or the vaccine is ineffective because the cold chain has been broken. Indicators to measure and evaluate process here would include checking appropriate cold chain conditions (measured through monitoring temperature) and the number of children receiving full courses of vaccine/number of ampoules used/number of syringes disposed of (usually measured on the basis of what is easiest/quickest or most reliable to collect). Clearly the context of the service delivery will affect this. In healthcare, a process represents the activities that constitute it and these include diagnosis, treatment, prevention, patient education and rehabilitation (Donabedian, 2003). These are usually carried out by doctors and healthcare professionals, although other contributors can include patients themselves and their families.

Evaluation of outcomes

This asks what type of effect the service is having on the users as well as on others who are involved in the service (staff, for instance). In healthcare speak, these are taken to mean changes – both desirable and undesirable – in both persons and populations that can be attributed to healthcare. Obvious changes are changes in health status. However there may be changes in knowledge acquired by patients and their next of kin that affect their behaviour. This in turn may influence future care and health, or indeed the satisfaction of patients with the care they received (Donabedian, 2003).

Evaluation of efficiency

Evaluation of outcomes asks if the service is benefitting the users and other stakeholders, evaluation of efficiency asks how these benefits compare with the costs of running the service. *Care pathways are altered, and commissioning decisions made, with the intention of benefitting patients, but often without fully understanding the cost implications. Using diabetes as an illustration, the briefing shows how organisations can use nationally available data to chart spending at a high level for various conditions* **www.audit-commission.gov.uk/SiteCollectionDocuments/Downloads/201105costofcarepathways.pdf**

There is a logical relationship between all of the above types of evaluation. Posovac and Carey in 1997 (cited by Robson, 2000, p49) stated that:

> *without measuring need, planning cannot be rational; without effective implementation, good outcomes cannot be expected; and without achieving good outcomes, there is no reason to worry about efficiency.*

Earlier aspects of an evaluation should be addressed first so that the later aspects of evaluation become relevant, although this does not always happen in reality. Changes may be prompted for external reasons (such as an alteration of government policy, unanticipated expenditure or the resignation of a key individual). People respond in the best way they can to immediate and pressing demands without sequential evaluation taking place. However, where planned change is to be successful, the steps described in the following section do need to be followed.

How to do a health service evaluation: basic stages and guidance

Health service evaluation proceeds through similar stages to any other kind of research – the differences lie in the detail. Activity 10.2 is intended to get you into the frame of mind for making sense of the guidance that follows.

ACTIVITY 10.2

Imagine you are planning to give a teaching session for a small group of second-year medical students on how to perform venepuncture using synthetic models in a clinical skills lab. You think it's a good idea to have your teaching session evaluated because you plan to do it again.

- What would you be interested to evaluate about your session?
- Who could you ask?
- How would you go about doing this? Give a basic step-by-step description of the stages you would go through to get a meaningful end result.
- What tools could you use to collect your data?

The steps you would go through to get a meaningful result are:

1. selecting the focus of review;

2. collecting appropriate information;

3. analysing the information;

4. interpreting and using the information;

5. reporting on activities and outcomes.

In this section, we will begin to link these 'building blocks' of knowledge together in a coherent way to construct an evaluation design.

Preparation stage

Do you really need to conduct an evaluation? Good evaluation takes time and costs resources, so this is a relevant question. Activity 10.3 suggests how you might decide the answer to this question.

ACTIVITY 10.3

Imagine you are a new Foundation year 1 doctor who has just started working for a respiratory consultant who runs the lung cancer multidisciplinary team (MDT) meetings. Someone mentions that it might be useful to find out how well the lung cancer specialist nurse service is supporting patients with lung cancer. Before you launch into planning an evaluation of this, can you think of anything you need to find out first that might help you decide if your own evaluation is needed or not?

Clue: Look up LUCADA on an internet search engine, and explore the webpages.

The possible case against conducting an evaluation in the activity above includes the following.

- Has the question already been answered? Has someone else done a similar project before you? Is there a national database to which your local MDT is already contributing? You may find that in many clinical specialties there is established support for service improvement using audit pathways (Chapter 9).

- Is there already generalisable research data/literature review to answer your query?

The possible case for conducting an evaluation in the activity above includes:

- Importance to patient welfare: is failure in care a frequent occurrence? Does it have serious consequences for health, or can any errors be corrected relatively easily?

- Is it high on the NHS priority list, e.g. dementia care?

- Is there pressure from politicians, patients or the public for better local care for this condition?

- Is expanding the service being considered?

- Has the service newly opened?

Even if an evaluation is needed, whether you go ahead depends on a few factors.

- Utility – are the evaluation results going to be useful and used?

- Feasibility – can something worthwhile be done within the time and resources available?

- Propriety – are there ethical aspects that need to be properly covered?

- Accuracy – will you be able to provide adequate and accurate information so that judgements can be made about the service? This information may be quantitative or qualitative; it may exist already or you may need to collect it.

These are interrelated with steps further downstream which will be discussed in more detail next. Activity 10.4 places this rather abstract set of guiding principles into a context. Comments under various stages will relate to the paper you first met in Activity 10.1. This close review of the paper – albeit for a different purpose – is like the review you would do when critically appraising a paper.

ACTIVITY 10.4

If you have not already done so, download: Ahmad *et al.* (2011). The impact of twice-daily consultant ward rounds on the length of stay in two general medical wards. *Clinical Medicine*, 11 (6): 524–8 **www.ingentaconnect.com/content/rcop/cm/2011/00000011/00000006/art00005**.

For each of the following steps, look at how the article reports what this study did. What was not considered (or reported)? Could/should anything you find missing have been considered? Compare your thoughts with ours.

Consult and involve help from stakeholders

As part of the preparation stage, you need to consider how you involve others. Involving others is a need, not a luxury! Stakeholder involvement is central to good evaluation. The need for others' involvement comes in a number of important ways. For example, others can help you by defining and refining the evaluation questions. Other advantages of involving others include getting help in gaining access and resources for evaluation, and optimising the impact of your evaluation results.

Issues which you should work through include:

- who are the stakeholders?

- the level of stakeholder involvement;

- service user motivation and support;

- persuading practitioners to get involved;

- vulnerable and/or hard-to-reach groups

Look back at Activity 10.1, where you listed people who have an interest in the change from twice-weekly to twice-daily ward rounds. Apart from hospital management and the consultants, did you include other ward staff in different roles, patients, carers of patients? In general, key stakeholders typically include:

- policy-makers and decision-makers;

- sponsors – people or organisations which have a funding or setting-up role;

- management;

- staff – people responsible for the delivery of service, e.g. doctors, nurses or supporting staff;

- clients/service users/patients;

- interested others – people who are geographically or politically 'close', e.g. patients' families, local politicians.

In practice the stakeholders most directly involved would be the sponsors (as they are funding the service), staff and management (as their performance is likely to come under scrutiny) and users (as they will be affected by the service). Therefore by encouraging active involvement of these stakeholders in focusing and designing the evaluation, you will be likely to make your evaluation useful. Pick out the stakeholders you feel are important for your evaluation, and decide their level of influence in the service. For those with intrinsically lower influence, you may have to think of ways to help get them more involved and increase that influence.

Case study: Stakeholders

In Liverpool, discussions with the consultants and other team members took place before the consultant-led ward rounds became twice daily. You can see in the acknowledgements at the end of the article that the diabetes and management team at the Royal Liverpool University Hospital were thanked for their hard work and the medical director supported the research (Ahmad *et al.*, 2011, p527).

The level of stakeholder involvement

Once you have decided on your key stakeholders, the next question is to what degree and how practically you are going to involve them. Examples include fellow evaluators, active responders or 'evaluation objects'. See Chapter 4 for more indepth discussion of each of these.

Service user motivation and support

You may also need to convince people to be involved in the evaluation. Consider what may motivate people to get involved; the ways service users could get involved and their level of responsibility; and how they will get feedback. Feedback is important not only as a check on how well you have understood their input but also to keep service users feeling part of the process. Be mindful of any specific issues (verbal reports for those unable to read, for instance) which may need to be addressed for different groups.

You may want to create a steering group that would have oversight of the logistics of such a stakeholder evaluation. Preparing people for participation is a part of the process (along with gaining resources and permissions). You cannot assume everyone will understand the nature of their role in the investigation. Training and ongoing support may be needed. An example of how this can be done is given below.

What's the evidence?

Involving beneficiaries

The extract that follows is from an article that reviews experience of engaging vulnerable people in the research process. A UK-wide research project aiming to improve interprofessional working in intermediate care teams wanted to recruit older people on to the research steering group.

> We believed it was important to actively involve clients and their carers in the development and direction of the research, because of their ability to provide insight concerning the realities of aging and accessing services, providing a perspective that could inform the research and address issues of importance to them as service users ... The research steering group included older people and carers, academics, practitioners of health and social care, and representatives from the voluntary sector; all were seen and treated as equal members of the group.
>
> To ensure that contributions were meaningful, a number of things had to be in place to facilitate involvement and to make sure that the older users and carers truly participated in the shaping and direction of the research. Members of an independent voluntary organization approached older users and carers, on the principal researcher's behalf, and invited them to participate in this research project; those who chose to participate in the research project were supported by a member of staff from the voluntary organization, with assistance and training from a research assistant from the research project. The users and carers were provided with training by one of the research assistants, which prepared them for their role prior to the commencement of the research. The preparatory training was staged, in line with progression of the research, and included an explanation of terminology associated with the subject, the research process itself, and information around technology support. All meetings were supported by the independent facilitator and researcher. By adopting this strategy, the users and carers were able to develop an understanding of the research approach and methodology, as well as to clarify understanding to apply their expertise that informed and directed the research.
>
> (Read and Maslin-Prothero, 2011, p707)

This extract shows that it is not sufficient simply to invite people to participate: you may also have to train and support them to make their contribution to an evaluation.

Vulnerable and/or hard-to-reach groups

Stakeholder involvement needs care and attention, particularly when vulnerable and/or hard-to-reach groups are involved. Examples include children, the homeless, asylum seekers and elderly patients. Be mindful of any specific issues which may need to be addressed for these groups.

Case study continued

Returning to the Liverpool study, what effect do you think the increase in earlier discharges had on the patients, their families, their carers and the wider community? We do not know if they were consulted in any way because we are not told. Whilst undoubtedly many patients would welcome earlier discharge, we cannot tell what the impact of that might be on support services where they live. Matters relating to patients were considered, however, in that outcomes (increased discharge rates, readmission rates and mortality) were measured, and no detrimental effect of the change was observed over a 12-month period.

Identifying, accessing and developing expertise

Do not be afraid to acknowledge your limitations, and do seek out support from those who can help you. You may need to learn new skills (which is a personally good reason for seeking to improve the quality of clinical care).

Case study continued

In Liverpool the professor of statistics provided his advice and guidance on statistical analysis to the researchers. The divisional analyst at the corporate information department provided the data and the medical director also supported the research (Ahmad *et al.*, 2011, p527).

Stage 1: Define your objective

An objective is the change that will be brought about as a result of your intervention. We have already looked at the importance of having clear objectives in order to focus your evaluation. You may have to prioritise these because of constraints of time, cost and resources. Objectives should be clear and specific, measurable, achievable, relevant and timely (SMART).

Table 10.1 outlines the relationship between reasons for evaluating and the types of questions to be asked.

Table 10.1 Reasons for evaluating

To find out if user needs are met	*To improve the programme*	*To assess outcomes of a programme*	*To find out how a programme is operating*	*To assess the efficiency of a programme*
Are we meeting the needs of our users/ patients?	How can we improve the service/ programme?	What happens to our users/patients as a result of participating in the service/programme?	What is actually going on during the running of a service/programme?	Are we making the best use of our resources in delivering this service/programme?
Are clinicians getting results in time to help with diagnosis?	Are patients satisfied with the service they are getting?	Does more rapid diagnosis improve patient care? Does it meet contractual obligations?	What constraints do service workers face?	What is the optimum throughput of processing of blood samples?

For a health service evaluation you should choose a relevant practice-based problem which could lead to tangible and useful ideas. Search for what is known already using PICO (patient/problem, intervention/exposure, comparison and outcome: Chapter 2).

Case study continued

In the evaluation we have been reviewing, activities were sparked because a variety of trust initiatives to reduce ALoS and increase safe discharges had already been tried in Liverpool. Two performance reviews and an audit had shown no benefit, so another approach was tried. The hypothesis tested by Ahmad *et al.* (2011) is stated in the methods section. The Liverpool research objective was to test the hypothesis that twice-daily consultant ward rounds would improve discharge planning, leading to an increased number of discharges and reducing ALoS with little impact, or potentially even an improvement, on the 28-day readmission rate and mortality (Ahmad *et al.*, 2011, p524).

Stage 2: Collect appropriate information

The next stage in the evaluation process is to collect appropriate information. When doing so, you need to consider the following questions.

- What study design will answer your question?

- What data will you collect, from whom and how?

- How will you analyse the data?

We will now look at each of these in turn.

What study design will answer your question?

Think about what you learned in Chapters 1 and 4.

Case study continued

The Liverpool study's quantitative study design compared the performance of two medical wards with the intervention (a twice-daily ward round which was provided by reorganising the work schedules of four consultants) with that of two other wards with a similar case load where consultants continued with twice-weekly ward rounds. The comparison took place over a year. The researchers also compared this with the baseline performance of all four wards in the previous year. It is not stated who the four consultants were – were they the authors of the publication?

The reading you did in Chapter 4 about action research makes this last point relevant. It's easier to change your own behaviour and that of like-minded colleagues than it is to persuade other people to change. The action research approach is very suitable for both health service evaluation and quality improvement where organisational change is intended. If this is a mixed-method approach, the interpretation of the results of the experimental design should take this into account.

What data will you collect, from whom and how?

Having formed a list of evaluation questions (based on your hypothesis and study design), you will need to consider what data to collect, from whom and how, and also how you can get trustworthy answers to your questions. Your evaluation objective is central to the design process and significantly determines the sampling strategy and methods. This should not be the other way around, however tempting the use of a particular method (see Chapters 1 and 4).

Case study continued

The evaluators used relevant routinely collected data from the hospital clinical information department from all four wards. The outcome variables measured were increased discharge rates, readmission rates and mortality, all of which were retrieved from routinely collected hospital data. It is implied that impact on costs and staff time were monitored, although it is not stated how this was done.

How will you analyse the data?

Finally you need to consider how you are going to analyse your data. This information is given in the final lines of the methods section of your report (and is covered in Chapter 6).

Case study continued

The evaluation analysed the quantitative data statistically and reported it in Table 1 (p525), which details the effects of twice-daily consultant ward rounds on the key measures, comparing the data on the wards before and after the change as well as comparing with the other medical wards where consultants continued with twice-weekly ward rounds.

Multimethod evaluation

Whatever tools you choose to employ to collect your information, the quality of data is always of paramount concern. Any single method will have its strengths and weaknesses. You may consider multimethod evaluation to optimise data quality, as illustrated by the National Child Measurement Programme (NCMP) report in Activity 10.5.

Activity 10.5 invites you to consider a different type of health service evaluation.

ACTIVITY 10.5

The NCMP is an important element of the government's programme on childhood obesity, and was launched in 2005. This joint initiative by the Departments of Health and Education involves measuring the weight and height of school children in Reception and Year 6 to inform local service planning and allow analysis of population trends in growth pattern and obesity.

Look up the Department of Health website (**www.dh.gov.uk**) and search for the report: 'A rapid review of the National Child Measurement Programme'.

- What were the purposes of the review?
- What were the methods of data collection?
- What were its main findings?

This six-week study considered *how well the NCMP is working, the challenges it faces and how it can be improved, particularly in light of the new public health arrangements within which the programme will in the future be operating* (Statham *et al.*, 2011, p50). The focus of the review was on the delivery of the NCMP rather than its impact on children and families. The study design is multimethod: data comprised documentary analysis, interviews with 17 key stakeholders and an online survey completed by 200 NCMP local leads and other relevant professionals. It was seen to have raised the profile of childhood obesity through providing evidence of its scale in England. However, challenges of funding and capacity meant there was considerable variability in how far local areas were able to provide routine feedback to parents about their child and to provide proactive follow-up.

Be realistic

In the collecting information stage, it is important to be realistic. As resources are generally limited, you must define the boundaries of your evaluation, which should include:

- timescale;

- people (their role and their time commitment);

- available finances;

- efficiency – maximum output with minimum input by using existing data, combining efforts with others and timing your evaluation for greatest likelihood of cooperation.

Stage 3: Interpreting and using the information

The next stage in the evaluation process is to interpret and use the information you have collected. Chapters 5 and 7 give guidance for this process in relation to research generally, but as health service evaluation seeks to improve healthcare you will want to identify the following.

- Who is the target audience?

- What form of evidence will convince and how does one make the evidence more credible?

The above questions are important because effective evaluation should convert into action for change. You will need to lay some foundations for success. To present the evaluation results more convincingly, you will have to know if your target audience responds to quantitative (numerical-based) or qualitative results (descriptive, e.g. quotations from 'real' voices of 'real' people) or a balance of both. This may partly influence the methods of data collection.

Case study continued

The quantitative research design is credible for convincing a target audience of hospital administrators and consultants about the success of the intervention. They interpreted the results in a context of economic recession thus:

> This study suggests that a cultural and behavioural shift in consultant working patterns can be achieved through innovative job planning, without increasing working hours or using extra resources. This system is sustainable and could possibly be replicated on medical wards with a mixed caseload of medical admissions. In the current financial environment, where excellent quality of care has to be provided with limited resources, new and innovative ways of working have to be devised, implemented and shared between trusts.
>
> (Ahmad et al., 2011, p527)

As mentioned before, to optimise the implementation of findings, the results need to be timely. Involvement of patient groups in healthcare settings, e.g. in dissemination of evaluation results, may also improve the likelihood of evaluation resulting in action, which is why communicating your results matters. This will be considered next.

Stage 4: Reporting and communicating the results

The next stage in the evaluation process is to report on and communicate the evaluation results. There are a variety of ways to do this:

- written reports;
- oral presentations, e.g. meetings, case studies;
- visual presentations, e.g. posters, web pages;
- existing literature, e.g. newsletters.

There may be more than one audience who needs to be informed. Any form of communication should be tailored to the target audience and the type of evidence they are likely to respond to. Issues relating to dissemination of results were discussed in Chapter 8.

Stage 5: Implementing change

The final stage in the evaluation process is to make a positive change happen as a result of the evaluation. How can we use the results of a service evaluation to improve care? The challenges in making appropriate changes are social and managerial (and political). Consequently it is generally senior staff who initiate change (even though their juniors implement it). However, it is worth remembering that health service evaluation is not to 'make work' but is the basis for making improvements. The World Health Organization (2003) lists practical routes to encourage change to improve the quality of healthcare service:

- information and communication – such as performance feedback;
- staff support – educational or training activities; incentives to motivate improvement; avoiding the blame culture;
- systems – provision of resources; restructuring and re-engineering towards patient needs;
- public involvement – gaining support for change through consultation.

Commonly used and useful management tools for promoting organisational change are well explained on the NHS Institute for Innovation and Improvement's website: **www.institute.nhs.uk/no_delays/introduction/fundamentals_for_ quality_improvement.html**

The basics of quality improvement

So far we have shown how clinical audit and health service evaluation can improve the delivery of healthcare in a variety of ways. Health service evaluation is linked to quality assurance and health improvement. Donabedian (2003, pxxiii) defines quality assurance as *all actions taken to establish, protect, promote, and improve the quality of healthcare*. In the UK, the term 'clinical governance' encompasses the philosophy of healthcare quality assurance, and has become entrenched in the working ethos of the NHS (Chapter 9).

The jigsaw of quality improvement also includes activities like audit, clinical incident reporting, risk management, appraisal and revalidation of healthcare professionals and so forth. The World Health Organization identified four components of quality which formed the basis of clinical governance in the NHS and underpinned Lord Darzi's White Paper *High Quality Care for All*, published in 2008 (Maybin and Thorlby, 2008). They are:

- professional performance and clinical effectiveness;

- resource use (efficiency);

- risk management (risk of injury or illness associated with the service provided) and patient safety;

- patient experience of the service.

This is how quality improvement stands today but the following 'What's the evidence?' shows the purposeful history from which it grew.

What's the evidence?

An abridged history of quality improvement and its antecedents

In Vienna in 1847 a doctor named Semmelweis *noted that puerperal fever was more common on a maternity ward where medical students worked than it was on the ward where midwives provided care* (Jarvis, 1994, p1311). His deduction that infection was transmitted by living organisms, and could be reduced by hand-washing with chlorinated lime, was not believed by his colleagues, although he repeatedly demonstrated success.

Systematic evaluation mainly undertaken by social scientists, using applied social research methods, mushroomed in the twentieth century (Rossi *et al.*, 2004). Evaluation was conducted for military programmes and policies in the USA during World War II. Rising expenditure on urban development, vocational and professional training and public health initiatives meant that interventions were expected to be evaluated and justified by success.

Healthcare services in the UK grew piecemeal following the establishment of the NHS in 1948, although services were largely unevaluated until the 1970s. Judging the effectiveness of an intervention means a comparison has to be made between those who receive the intervention and a control group (people with similar characteristics) who do not. People are randomly assigned to one group or the other but many felt having a comparison group where some individuals are not offered services was unethical. In the 1960s, when Archie Cochrane directed the Medical Research Council Epidemiology Unit in Cardiff, many people resisted the idea of conducting randomised controlled trials (Cochrane and Blythe, 1989).

Gradually, evaluation became driven by the stakeholders of evaluation: policy-makers, administrators, programme organisers and those affected by these interventions (the public, funding bodies, and so on). Maxwell reported that, following exposure of cruel and inhumane treatment of 'mentally retarded' patients in a hospital in Ely, UK in the 1970s:

---

the Hospital Advisory Service . . . [set up by Richard Crossman in 1969] was intended to be his eyes and ears in the long stay sector. This was in the wake of a series of incidents and inquiries, such as that at Ely. Multidisciplinary teams visit the major long stay institutions to examine standards of care, and recommend improvements when appropriate. The teams discuss their findings on the spot, and make a written report to the district health authority and to the Secretary of State.

(Maxwell, 1984, p1470)

The Armenian physician Avedis Donabedian (1919–2000) influenced the development of the concept of quality assurance and monitoring in healthcare. His 1966 seminal work 'Evaluating the quality of medical care' made the now classic distinction between structure, process and outcome. This recognises how quality depends on many components and that process and outcome can be assessed separately. In 1984 Maxwell identified six core dimensions of quality: cost, equity, humanity, relevance to need, social acceptability and technical excellence.

From the mid-1990s the issue of patient safety emerged exponentially, following observations (initially in the USA) of widespread variations in the quality of care across different geographical areas. Publication of the US Institute of Medicine's 1999 report *To Err is Human* galvanised professional and political concern with improving patient safety (Kohn *et al.*, 2000). The UK equivalent was *An Organisation with a Memory* (Department of Health, 2000).

Don Berwick, drawing inspiration from managerial techniques developed in hazardous industries (aviation and the nuclear industry, for example) as well as Japanese car companies, placed emphasis on the process of learning from mistakes, and designing failsafe processes into systems (Vincent, 2010). This is why an inquiry chaired by Robert Francis QC was set up in June 2010 to find out why serious problems at the Mid Staffordshire NHS Foundation Trust were not identified and acted on sooner and to identify important lessons to be learnt for the future of patient care (**www. midstaffspublicinquiry.com**). Relevant commissioning, supervisory and regulatory organisations have submitted reports regarding their monitoring role at the trust between January 2005 and March 2009. The inquiry hearings concluded on 1 December 2011, and it has now adjourned for the Chairman to write his final report.

Concerns about mortality and the standard of care provided at Stafford Hospital resulted in an investigation by the Healthcare Commission which published a highly critical report in March 2009. This was followed by two reviews commissioned by the Department of Health. These investigations gave rise to widespread public concern and a loss of confidence in the trust, its services and management. The first Robert Francis QC Inquiry report into the care provided by Mid Staffordshire NHS Foundation Trust was published in March 2010. Based on evidence submitted by over 900 patients and families, it reported that patients were routinely neglected by a trust preoccupied with cost cutting, targets and processes. It had lost sight of its fundamental responsibility to provide safe care. Chronic staff shortages, particularly of nursing staff, mainly accounted for the substandard care. Morale at the trust was low, and, while many staff did their best under difficult circumstances, others showed a disturbing lack of compassion towards their patients. Staff who spoke out felt ignored, and there was strong evidence that many were silenced through fear and bullying (**www.midstaffsinquiry.com**).

Since then clinical quality review meetings (CQRMs) have become well established with the main providers: University Hospital North Staffordshire; North Staffordshire Combined Health Care; North Staffordshire Community Health services; and Stoke-on-Trent Community Health Services. The CQRMs are mandated as part of the national contract and provide the central hub for monitoring the quality and safety of services commissioned.

Meanwhile the University Hospital of North Staffordshire has published detailed annual Quality Accounts since 2009–10 that are online. It has won entries in the NHS Institute Patient Safety Awards and the Lean Academy Awards.

Today, campaigns such as 1000 Lives stem from the Institute for Healthcare Improvement (**www.ihi.org/Pages/default.aspx**). Healthcare students have a key role to play in improving patient safety and healthcare quality improvement. With an awareness of quality improvement and patient safety, the NHS workforce of the future is vital to sustaining cultural change.

Why safety matters and how it is promoted

One in ten patients will suffer an adverse event when they are hospitalised. This shocking statistic of avoidable harm could be reduced by prioritising patient safety when designing processes, equipment, organisational systems and working practices. Vincent (2010) describes how concern with patient safety represents a confluence of ideas from a number of different fields. Improving the quality of care (as shown in the above 'What's the evidence?') has been shaped by changes in the nature of error, as the following quotation indicates.

> *To learn only from one's own mistakes would be a slow and painful process and unnecessarily costly to one's patients. Experiences need to be pooled so that doctors may also learn from the errors of others. This requires a willingness to admit that one has erred and to discuss the factors that may have been responsible. It calls for a critical attitude to one's own work and to that of others. Unfortunately medical students and doctors see little evidence of such openness around them.*
>
> (McIntyre and Popper, 1983, p1919)

Among all other professionals, doctors have enormous responsibility and are held to account. We learn to start assuming responsibility for other people, essentially strangers, from the time we are students. Whether it is to give a drug, operate or oversee the delivery of a service, we learn early on that there are competencies, standards, but most of all a sense of responsibility to our patients. Quality assurance and patient safety should really be regarded as a touchstone that we are doing everything in our power to keep our patients out of harm's way and improve the way they are looked after. It is incumbent on the system we work in that we evaluate the way we work and the outcome for our patients but it is inherent in the way doctors train that they do everything they can to make life (and the end of life) as comfortable for the patients as they can. This is worth remembering while we feel the microscope of evaluation upon us. Organisations are just watching what most of us are committed to doing without needing to be asked.

Further stimuli to improve quality of care come from examples of practices in high-risk industries such as the nuclear and aviation industries. Recognition that human error is inevitable (through tiredness, inexperience or momentary inattention, for example, or psychological 'force of habit') and pressure from government and the public together with litigation from patients in response to a number of high-profile tragedies such as the Bristol (**www.bristol-inquiry.org.uk**), Shipman (**www.shipman-inquiry.org.uk/home.asp**) and Alder Hey (**www. rlcinquiry.org.uk/download/index.htm**) Inquiries have provided further impetus for the medical profession.

The response in the UK has been to encourage healthcare organisations to become learning organisations. Learning happens through reporting not only 'adverse incidents' (those that resulted in harm, whether they arose from an error or could not be prevented, such as very low birth weight) but also 'near misses' and reflecting on the actions taken and what could have been done differently. Reviewing processes to see where there is potential for error reduction to be 'designed out' enables all staff to contribute to the process.

Patient safety is *The avoidance, prevention and amelioration of adverse outcomes or injuries stemming from the process of healthcare* (Vincent, 2010, p31). Delivering healthcare to patients is a hospital's priority. Safety is balanced against other aspects of the quality of care in a context of resource and cost constraints. Clinicians discuss risky but potentially curative therapies with a patient who in turn balances the risk against other matters of importance (being able to lift his grandson, for instance). As a final activity, Activity 10.6 encourages you to think what your own contribution to promoting quality improvement might be.

ACTIVITY 10.6

Read the third-year student blog on the Institute for Healthcare Improvement site: **www.ihiopenschool.blogspot.com/2012/01/dont-be-that-guy-tips-from-third-year.html**

Add your own contribution.

Improving quality is not just about how you interact with others (the starting point of that blog), although that is clearly important. Improving quality means taking personal responsibility and acting whenever it is feasible to do so.

Chapter summary

- Evaluation is the assessment and determination of the quality or value of something.

- The purpose of evaluation is to see what changes need to be made (and sometimes, whether something should continue) and then making them.

- Evaluation of healthcare services looks at structure, process, outcomes, efficiency, value for money, equity and humanity.

- The stages of evaluation are: selecting the focus of review; collecting appropriate information; analysing the information; interpreting and using the information; reporting on activities and outcomes.

- Evaluation involves all the stakeholders, although there may be differences in when and how they become involved.

- Evaluation for high-quality care involves professional performance and clinical effectiveness; resource use (efficiency); risk management (risk of injury or illness associated with the service provided) and patient safety; and patient experience of the service.

- Quality improvement involves not only evaluation but action and learning, and so employs a variety of managerial techniques.

- Patient safety is *The avoidance, prevention and amelioration of adverse outcomes or injuries stemming from the process of healthcare* (Vincent, 2010, p31).

GOING FURTHER

Clinical Skills Unit (2006) University of Cambridge/Addenbrooke's NHS Cascading Teaching Communication Skills Website Trust. **www.commscascade.med-schl.cam.ac.uk**
Some excellent learning materials relating to communication skills.

Darzi, A (2008) *A High Quality Workforce: NHS next stage review.* London: Department of Health.
An influential policy document.

Jarvis, WR (1994) Handwashing – the Semmelweis lesson forgotten? *Lancet* 344 (8933): 1311–12. *Fascinating account of Semmelweis' experiments with his medical students, and how the problem of hand-washing remains to be solved.*

McKimm, J and Forrest, K (eds) (2011) *Professional Practice for Foundation Doctors.* Exeter: Learning Matters.

Marsh, P and Glendenning, R (2005) *Primary Care Service Evaluation Toolkit.* **www.camstrad.nhs.uk/documents/Researchers/evaluation_toolkit. pdf?preventCache=08/08/2005%2015:16**
This resource offers clear step-by-step practical guidance on how to conduct a service evaluation.

National Health Service Institute for Innovation and Improvement (2008) *Fundamentals for Quality Improvement.* **www.institute.nhs.uk/no_delays/ introduction/fundamentals_for_quality_improvement.html**
A variety of useful management tools to improve healthcare quality.

Ritti, RR and Levy, S (2010) *The Ropes to Skip and the Ropes to Know*: *Studies in organisational theory and behaviour,* 8th edition. Chichester: John Wiley.
Described as 'the instruction manual to your corporate career', this is a highly readable book explaining the tacit features of organisational behaviour. You'll gain critical insights into human interaction and power from this very entertainingly written book.

Vincent, C (2010) *Patient Safety,* 2nd edition. Oxford: Wiley-Blackwell.
A comprehensive textbook on this important topic.

National Health Service Institute for Innovation and Improvement: **www.institute. nhs.uk**
A web portal to bookmark.

DIPEx: **www.healthtalkonline.org**
A database of over 2,000 people's experiences of illness, covering a wide range of diseases and health problems using text, audio and visual clips. These are based on qualitative research led by Oxford University experts.

Glossary

Association A possible co-occurrence or relationship between two variables. Does not mean a cause-and-effect relationship has been established.

Benchmark The management process whereby organisations evaluate various aspects of their processes in relation to the best practice, usually within their own sector.

Beneficence The moral principle of doing good.

Case-control study A type of observational analytic epidemiological investigation in which subjects are selected on the basis of whether they do (cases) or do not (controls) have a particular disease. The groups are then compared with respect to the proportion having a history of exposure or characteristic of interest.

Case series A series of patients with a defined disorder. The term is used to describe a study reporting on a consecutive collection of patients treated in a similar manner, without a concurrent control group. For example, a surgeon might describe the characteristics of and outcomes for 100 consecutive patients with cerebral ischaemia who received a revascularisation procedure.

Clinical governance Chapter 6 of the 1997 White Paper *The New NHS: Modern, dependable* (Department of Health, 1997) described the means of improving clinical standards at local level throughout the NHS. It involves:

- action to ensure that risks are avoided;
- rapid detection of adverse events which are openly investigated and lessons learned;
- disseminating good practice;
- establishing systems to ensure continuous improvements in clinical care.

Clinical governance is the system through which NHS organisations are accountable for continuously improving the quality of their services and safeguarding high standards of care, by creating an environment in which clinical excellence will flourish (Department of Health, 1998).

Clinical trial A prospective controlled study involving patients, i.e. one in which an intervention is allocated and patients are followed up.

Cluster trial An interventional design which attempts to make inferences about individuals but where the intervention is allocated to clusters of individuals.

Coding frame Coding is an analytical process in which data are categorised to facilitate analysis. One code should apply to only one category and categories should be comprehensive. The coding framework is the clear guidelines for coders (individuals who do the coding) to ensure that code is consistently applied.

Cohort A group of individuals who share a characteristic (such as age, gender). In a cohort study, individuals are followed for a period of time to determine disease incidence at different ages.

Confounding variable A factor which is significantly associated with both the occurrence of a disease in a population and with one of the causes or determinants, but is not itself a cause. Confounding variables can result in erroneous conclusions. For example, vegetarians have a lower incidence of obesity than non-vegetarians, but the lower incidence of obesity may be due to the confounding factor that vegetarians tend to be more active as a population than non-vegetarians rather than the lower incidence being due to difference in diet.

Controlled experiment Research studies in which variables are controlled. Typically one group receives a treatment and another (the control group) does not. The groups are similar in every characteristic except for the treatment so that differences in the groups can be attributed to the treatment.

Conversation analysis A form of discourse analysis that studies social interaction, embracing both verbal and non-verbal conduct, in situations of everyday life.

Correlation A measure of the association between two or more variables. The measurement scales used should be at least interval. Correlation is not causation but it may imply that link is worth further investigation. The most widely used type of correlation coefficient is Pearson r, also called linear or product moment correlation.

Cross-sectional A cross-sectional study is a descriptive study in which disease and exposure status are measured simultaneously in a given population. Such a study provides a snapshot of the frequency and characteristics of a disease in a population at a particular point in time.

Crowd-sourcing In the world of technology, crowd-sourcing means inviting a group to collaborate on a solution to a problem. It was coined by Jeff Howe of *Wired* magazine in 2006 to refer to *the widespread internet practice of posting an open call requesting help in completing some task.*

Data corpus The whole body of data collected.

Data matrix Another word for a table where data are entered into individual cells.

Data set The sample from a data corpus that you select for scrutiny for a particular purpose.

Deductive reasoning The process of arguing from a general to a specific instance (from a theory to an empirical situation, for instance).

Delphi technique With the Delphi technique, individual participants are asked to give their views in response to a series of questions. These views are collated and are then fed back to the participants, who rank them in order of importance to them. This second round is collated and fed back to all the participants again. This creates an opportunity for individuals to revise their judgements on the basis of this feedback and gives some degree of anonymity for their individual contributions. Although time-intensive and somewhat expensive, it is a useful tool for establishing a consensus about priorities relevant for a particular target group (such as elderly people or those with disabilities) who are most knowledgeable about their specific needs.

Discourse analysis A general term for a number of qualitative approaches to analysing written, spoken or signed language use.

Ecological fallacy This occurs when you extrapolate from group data to draw conclusions about individuals.

Effective How well a treatment works in practice (as opposed to the controlled conditions present in a clinical trial, where efficacy is measured).

Efficient/Efficiency An economics concept that relates to the optimal use of resources.

Emic perspective Description of behaviour or a belief in terms meaningful (consciously or unconsciously) to the person within the culture.

Empiricism A theory of knowledge that asserts that knowledge comes only or primarily via sensory experience.

Epidemiological The branch of medicine dealing with the study of the causes, distribution and control of disease in populations.

Epistemic community A network of professionals with recognised expertise and competence with an authoritative claim to knowledge within a particular area. Although an epistemic community may consist of professionals from a variety of disciplines and backgrounds, they have a shared set of normative and principled beliefs.

Equipoise When two treatments are regarded as an equal bet in prospective terms.

Ethnographic research A qualitative study design that entails indepth study of a society's or an organisation's culture and social structure. It uses both qualitative and quantitative methods to do this.

Evaluation The assessment and determination of the quality or value of something (for purposes both of accountability and for learning).

Evidence-based medicine Aims to apply the best available evidence gained from the scientific method to clinical practice.

Experimental A systematic testing process that is carried out in order to verify, falsify or establish the validity of a hypothesis.

Focus group A group interview where people who are strangers to each other but have experience of what is being investigated are invited to contribute their views and ideas. The hope is that as wide a range of differing opinions or experiences as possible will be expressed.

Formative evaluation Looks for areas for improvement in a service.

Generalisability This exists when the results of the research can be applied more generally and more widely than the research study itself.

Guidelines Any document that seeks to standardise processes associated with an activity and thus make employees' actions accountable. By definition, following a guideline is never mandatory. 'Protocol' would be a better term for a procedure that is mandatory. They are part of the wider process of governance. The National Library of Guidelines is a collection of guidelines for the NHS. It is based on the guidelines produced by NICE and other national agencies.

Hegemony (hegemonic) The predominant political economic and ideological influence (of a state, region or group) over others so that its way of seeing things is perceived as natural and common-sense.

Heterogeneity In systematic reviews, heterogeneity refers to variability or differences between studies in the estimates of effects.

Histogram A frequency distribution by means of rectangles whose widths represent class intervals and whose areas are proportional to the corresponding frequencies.

Implementation research *Implementation research is the scientific study of methods to promote the systematic uptake of clinical research findings and other evidence-based practices into routine practice, and hence to improve the quality (effectiveness, reliability, safety, appropriateness, equity, efficiency) of healthcare. It includes the study of influences on healthcare professional and organisational behaviour* (**www.who.int/reproductivehealth/topics/best_practices/greatproject_glossary/en/index.html**).

Inception cohort A designated group of persons, assembled at a common time early in the development of a specific clinical disorder (for example, at the time of first exposure to the putative (i.e. supposed) cause or at the time of initial diagnosis), who are followed thereafter.

Inductive reasoning The process of inference from a finite number of particular cases in order to make a generalisation.

Interpretivist This paradigm starts from the view that people construct meanings through language and interaction with others in their daily lives. Thus any attempt to establish cause-and-effect relationships is misguided because meanings will change in different situations and over time.

Intervention Any activity or object whose purpose is to improve health or alter the course of disease.

Interview Formal talk where questions are asked by the interviewer to obtain information from the respondent in order to collect data to answer the research question.

Interview schedule A formal list of precoded questions that must be asked in the same order and in the same way by an interviewer who writes down on it the answers given.

Key informant Anyone who can provide detailed information and opinion based on his or her knowledge of a particular issue.

Liberalism A set of ideas in political and social thought which underlines the importance of individual rights. The role of the state is primarily to protect these rights (referred to as neoliberalism when it includes market-driven ideas of the efficiency of private enterprise justifying the diminishment of the public sector).

Mainstreaming A process whereby an activity or idea becomes popularised or adopted as policy that attracts routine funding.

Mean The average where you add up all the numbers and then divide by the number of numbers.

Median Another form of average that is the numerical value separating the higher half of a sample (or population) from the lower half.

Meta-analysis The statistical analysis of data from more than one study of the same intervention (or association) in an attempt to summarise the current state of knowledge.

Mode Another measure of average that is the value that occurs most often.

Narrative review Discusses and summarises the literature on a particular topic, without generating any pooled summary figures through meta-analysis. This type of review usually gives a comprehensive overview of a topic, rather than addressing a specific question such as how effective a treatment is for a particular condition. Narrative reviews do not often report on how the search for literature was carried out or how it was decided which studies were relevant to include. Therefore, they are not classified as systematic reviews.

National Institute for Health and Clinical Excellence (NICE) Provides guidance, sets quality standards and manages a national database to improve people's health and prevent and treat ill health. It uses research evidence as well as economic information and consultation with service users for policy-making.

Nominal group A group interview where the aim is to establish consensus about the issue being investigated. Nominal group technique is a structured method for group brainstorming that encourages contributions from everyone.

Non-maleficence The moral principle of not doing harm. It is one of the four principles in medical ethics proposed by Beauchamp and Childress (2001).

Null hypothesis The proposition to be tested statistically, that the experimental intervention has 'no effect'.

Nuremberg Code In 1947 an international tribunal declared the Nuremberg Code the standard by which a group of doctors in Nazi Germany should be judged.

Odds ratio One of a range of statistics used to assess the risk of a particular outcome (or disease) if a certain factor (or exposure) is present.

Outcome Something that follows as a result or consequence of an intervention. Measurable outcomes need to be specified as a part of the design of evaluation research. They are the higher-level results.

Paradigm A shared stable commitment to key theories, instruments, values and underpinning assumptions that form the discipline, thus facilitating the cumulative generation of knowledge. It was a concept used by Thomas Kuhn in *The Structure of Scientific Revolutions* (1962).

Performance framework Following on from the 1997 White Paper *The New NHS: Modern, dependable* (Department of Health, 1997), NHS trusts became required to report on the following six areas:

1. health improvement;

2. fair access to services;

3. effective delivery of appropriate healthcare;

4. efficiency;

5. patient/carer experience;

6. the health outcomes of NHS care.

Phenomenology A world view that values the meaning of occurrences, rather than measuring observable events.

Placebo A chemically inert substance which has a psychologically suggestive effect and is used in place of an active drug. It may be used as a control in a clinical trial to determine whether improvement and/or side effects can be attributed to the active substance.

Positivist A world view that values measurement and observable events.

Post-positivist A social science approach studying how people construct meaning through social interaction.

Power The power of a statistical hypothesis test measures the test's ability to reject the null hypothesis when it is actually false – in other words, to make a correct decision. It is the probability of not committing a type II error (failing to recognise a difference when in fact there is one – which can happen when a sample size is too small).

Process measures The activities that can be identified that feed into an outcome. They can be monitored to ensure work is on track to achieve its objectives.

Prospective A research design that follows respondents into the future (also called longitudinal).

Protocol A formal and explicit treatment regimen for care. A clinical trial will have two or more such protocols along with a description of the research design or method, eligibility requirements and the proposed method of analysis. It can also be used to describe the comprehensive written document detailing all procedures to be followed in a trial.

Publication bias A tendency to publish results that appear significant, rather than negative or near-neutral results, which are almost never published. This can distort the true picture of research findings if a meta-analysis is performed as the success of an intervention is overrepresented.

Q-squared (Q^2) methods Also known as mixed methods, Q-squared methods refer to a study design that incorporates both quantitative and qualitative methods. Data is analysed severally. Such an approach deepens understanding.

Qualitative research An approach that aims to form an indepth understanding of human behaviour and the reasons that govern such behaviour.

Quality Measures of excellence in either a service or product.

Randomised controlled trial (RCT) An epidemiological study where people are randomly allocated to receive (or not receive) a particular intervention (this could be two different treatments or one treatment and a placebo). This experimental study design is used to determine whether an intervention or treatment is more effective than the alternative control.

Relative risk Risk of an event (or of developing a disease) relative to exposure. Relative risk is a ratio of the probability of the event occurring in the exposed group versus a non-exposed group.

Reliable The consistency of a set of measurements or of a measuring tool (interview schedule, for example). Reliability is necessary but not sufficient for validity.

Representative The extent to which sample data reflect accurately the characteristics of the population from which they are drawn.

Retrospective study A study that examines events that have already taken place; a study on previously collected data.

Sampling frame A comprehensive list of names and contact details.

Selection bias A statistical bias that can arise through the method of choosing the individuals or groups to take part in a scientific study.

Social accountability Being mindful of the emerging social concerns and priorities of internal and external stakeholders (patients, community, employees, governmental and non-governmental organisations, management and owners).

Social constructivism A paradigm interested in how an individual's learning takes place because of his or her interactions in a group.

Stakeholder A person, group or organisation that has direct or indirect stake in an organisation because it can affect or be affected by the organisation's actions, objectives and policies.

Standards Both governance and quality issues. Organisations publish practical guidance and examples of good practice to which they wish employees to adhere and for which sanctions apply if they are not followed.

Structured questionnaires A series of questions asked to individuals to obtain statistically useful information about a given topic that may be posted to people/be online and so be self-completed, or may be asked by an interviewer (referred to as interview schedules).

Summative evaluation Forms a judgement of the value and merits of whatever is being evaluated, usually for decision-making and accountability purposes.

Survey Observational or descriptive, non-experimental study in which individuals are systematically examined for the absence or presence (or degree of presence) of characteristics of interest.

Synonyms Different words with almost identical or similar meanings – a thesaurus can be used to identify such words.

Systematic review A synthesis of medical research on a particular subject to represent the current stage of knowledge about what is effective clinical practice. It uses thorough methods to search for and include all or as much as possible of the research on the topic. Only relevant studies, usually of a certain minimum methodological quality, are included.

Transactions costs The resources needed (time, money, expertise, for example) to deliver a product or service. In healthcare this would include costs arising from different governance structures of local and health authorities when a patient's care entails crossing organisational boundaries.

Translational research or **implementation science** Promotes the uptake of research findings into routine healthcare in both clinical and policy contexts. It is multidisciplinary research that scientifically studies methods to promote the systematic uptake of clinical research findings and other evidence-based practices into routine practice, so as to improve the quality and effectiveness of healthcare. It includes the study of what influences healthcare professional and organisational behaviour.

Triangulation This involves using more than one method to produce different forms of data (or the same method to gather data from different sources). The data can be compared, and similar findings from different methods may support the validity and comprehensiveness of the research findings.

Type II error The false acceptance of the null hypothesis (a false negative). The type I error (false positive) is more serious: it wrongly rejects the null hypothesis.

Valid The metric corresponds accurately to what it claims to be occurring in the real world.

Variable The name given to a category that can change its value.

White Paper A White Paper issued by the government lays out policy, or intended action, on a topic that is of current concern. It signifies an intention to issue new law, and in the UK is also known as a Command paper. White Papers are often preceded by Green Papers, which are consultation documents.

References

The Academy of Medical Royal Colleges (2012) *Foundation Programme Curriculum 2012*. www.foundationprogramme.nhs.uk/pages/home

Acheson, D (1998) *Independent Inquiry into Inequalities in Health Report*. London: The Stationery Office.

Ahmad, A, Purewal, TS, Sharma, D and Weston, PJ (2011) The impact of twice-daily consultant ward rounds on the length of stay in two general medical wards. *Clinical Medicine*, 11(6): 524–8.

Anderson, MS and Steneck, NH (2011) The problem of plagiarism. *Urologic Oncology: Seminars and Original Investigations*, 29(1): 90–4.

Andersson, O, Hellström-Westas, L, Andersson, D and Domellöf, M (2011) Effect of delayed versus early umbilical cord clamping on neonatal outcomes and iron status at 4 months: a randomised controlled trial. *British Medical Journal*, 343: d7157.

Antithrombotic Trialists' Collaboration (2009) Aspirin in the primary and secondary prevention of vascular disease: collaborative meta-analysis of individual participant data from randomised trials. *Lancet*, 373(9678): 1849–60.

Atkin, K and Ahmad, W (2000) Pumping iron: compliance with chelation therapy among young people who have thalassaemia major. *Sociology of Health & Illness*, 22(4): 500–24.

Atkinson, JM and Heritage, J (eds) (1984) *Structures of Social Action: Studies in conversation analysis*. Cambridge: Cambridge University Press.

Attia, J and Page, J (2001) A graphic framework for teaching critical appraisal of randomised controlled trials. *Evidence Based Medicine*, 6(3): 68–9.

Bannerjee, S (2009) *The Use of Antipsychotic Medication for People with Dementia: Time for action*. www.dh.gov.uk/prod_consum_dh/groups/dh_digitalassets/documents/digitalasset/dh_108302.pdf

Barbour, RS (2001) Checklists for improving rigour in qualitative research: a case of the tail wagging the dog? *British Medical Journal*, 322(7294): 1115–17.

Bartley, M (2004) *Health Inequality: An introduction to theories, concepts and methods*. Cambridge: Polity Press/Blackwell Publishing.

Bashshur, R (ed.) (2003) *An Introduction to Quality Assurance in Health Care: Avedis Donabedian*. Oxford: Oxford University Press.

Basit, TN (2003) Manual or electronic? The role of coding in qualitative data analysis. *Educational Research,* 45(2): 143–54.

Beauchamp, TL and Childress, J (2001) *Principles of Biomedical Ethics* (5th edition). Oxford: Oxford University Press.

Becker, H (2007) *Writing for Social Scientists: How to start and finish your thesis, book or article.* Chicago, IL: University of Chicago Press.

Bohmer, R (2010) Leadership with a small "l". *British Medical Journal,* 340: 265.

Booth, A (2010) How much searching is enough? Comprehensive versus optimal retrieval for technology assessments. *International Journal of Technology Assessment in Health Care,* 26(4): 431–5.

Bowling, A and Ebrahim, S (2005) *Handbook of Health Research Methods: Investigation, measurement and analysis.* Maidenhead: Open University Press.

Brew, A (2007) Research and teaching from the students' perspective. International policies and practices for academic enquiry: an international colloquium held at Marwell Conference Centre, Winchester, UK, 19–21 April.

Broom, A, Cheshire, L and Emmison, M (2009) Qualitative researchers' understandings of their practice and the implications for data archiving and sharing. *Sociology,* 43(6): 1163–80.

Burgoyne, LN, O'Flynn, S and Boylan, GB (2010) Undergraduate medical research: the student perspective. *Medical Education Online,* 15: 5212.

Burns, E (2010) Developing email interview practices in qualitative research. *Sociological Research Online,* 15(4): 8

Buzan, T (1996) *The Mind Map Book.* Harmondsworth: Penguin Books.

Carthey, J, Walker, S, Deelchand, V, Vincent, C and Griffiths, WH (2011) Breaking the rules: understanding non-compliance with policies and guidelines. *British Medical Journal,* 343: 5283.

Cheesmond, AK and Fenwick, A (1981) Human excretion behaviour in a schistosomiasis endemic area of the Geizira, Sudan. *Transactions of the Royal Society of Tropical Medicine and Hygiene,* 84: 101–7.

Clinical Governance Support Team NHS (2005) *Practical Clinical Audit Handbook.* London: NHS.

Cochrane, AL (1972) *Effectiveness and Efficiency.* London: Nuffield Provincial Hospitals Trust.

Cochrane, AL and Blythe, M (1989) *One Man's Medicine.* London: British Medical Journal, 61–72.

Cohen, L, Manion, L and Morrison, K (2011) *Research Methods in Education,* 7th edition. Abingdon: Routledge.

Crombie, IK, Davies, HTO, Abraham, SCS and Florey, C du V (1993) *The Audit Handbook: Improving healthcare through clinical audit.* Chichester: John Wiley.

Curtis, V, Cousens, S, Mertens, T, Traore, E, Kanki, B and Diallo, I (1993) Structured observations of hygiene behaviours in Burkina Faso: validity, variability, and utility. *Bulletin of the World Health Organization,* 71(1): 23–32.

Dadich, A and Muir, K (2009) Tricks of the trade in community mental health research: working with mental health services and clients. *Evaluation & the Health Professions,* 32(1): 38–58.

Darzi, A (2008) Evidence-based medicine and the NHS: a commentary. *Journal of the Royal Society of Medicine,* 101(7): 342–4.

Das, K, Malick, S and Khan, KS (2008) Tips for teaching evidence-based medicine in a clinical setting: lessons from adult learning theory. Part one. *Journal of the Royal Society of Medicine,* 101(10): 493–500.

Davidson, EJ (2005) *Evaluation Methodology Basics: The nuts and bolts of sound evaluation.* London: Sage Publications.

de Salis, I, Tomlin, Z, Toerien, M and Donovan, J (2008) Qualitative research to improve RCT recruitment: issues arising in establishing research collaborations. *Contemporary Clinical Trials,* 29(5): 663–70.

Denzin, NK (2009) The elephant in the living room: or extending the conversation about the politics of evidence. *Qualitative Research* 9(2): 139–60.

Denzin, N and Lincoln, Y (1994) *Handbook of Qualitative Research.* London: Sage.

Department of Health (1989) *Working for Patients: Medical audit working paper no. 6.* London: HMSO.

Department of Health (1997) *The New NHS: Modern, dependable.* Cm 3807. London: The Stationery Office.

Department of Health (1998) *A First Class Service: Quality in the new NHS.* London: Department of Health.

Department of Health (2000) *An Organisation with a Memory: Report of an expert group on learning from adverse events in the NHS.* London: The Stationery Office.

Department of Health (2002) *Learning from Bristol: The report of the public inquiry into children's heart surgery at the Bristol Royal Infirmary 1984–1995.* Command paper CM 5363. London: The Stationery Office.

Department of Health (2005) *Research Governance Framework for Health and Social Care,* 2nd edition. www.dh.gov.uk/en/Publicationsandstatistics/Publications/PublicationsPolicyAndGuidance/DH_4108962.

Department of Health and Social Security (1980) Inequalities in health: report of a research working group (the Black report). London: DHSS.

Dixon, RA, Munro, JF and Silcocks, PB (eds) (1997) *The Evidence Based Medicine Workbook: Critical appraisal for evaluating clinical problem solving.* Oxford: Butterworth-Heinemann.

Dommeyer, CJ and Moriarty, E (2000) Comparing two forms of an e-mail survey: embedded vs. attached. *International Journal of Market Research*, 42(1): 39–50.

Donabedian, A (1966) Evaluating the quality of medical care. *The Milbank Memorial Fund Quarterly*, 44(3): 166–206.

Donabedian, A (1978) The quality of medical care. *Science*, 200(4344): 856–64.

Donabedian, A (2003) *An Introduction to Quality Assurance in Health Care.* New York: Oxford University Press.

Dowswell, G, Ismail, T, Greenfield, S, Clifford, S, Hancock, B and Wilson, S (2011) Men's experience of erectile dysfunction after treatment for colorectal cancer: qualitative interview study. *British Medical Journal*, 343: d5824.

Dunne, C (2011) The place of the literature review in grounded theory research. *International Journal of Social Research Methodology*, 14(2): 111–24.

Egan, K, Harcourt, D, Rumsey, N and Antithrombotic Trialists' Collaboration (2011) A qualitative study of the experiences of people who identify themselves as having adjusted positively to a visible difference. *Journal of Health Psychology*, 16(5): 739–49.

Ehrich, K, Williams, C and Farsides, B (2010) Fresh or frozen? Classifying 'spare' embryos for donation to human embryonic stem cell research. *Social Science & Medicine*, 71(12): 2204–11.

Finlay, L (2006) 'Rigour', 'ethical integrity' or 'artistry'? Reflexively reviewing criteria for evaluating qualitative research. *British Journal of Occupational Therapy*, 69(7): 319–26.

Garfinkel, H (1967) *Studies in Ethnomethodology.* New York: Prentice Hall.

Garner, J, McKendree, J, O'Sullivan, H and Taylor, D (2010) Undergraduate medical student attitudes to the peer assessment of professional behaviours in two medical schools. *Education for Primary Care*, 21(1): 32–7.

General Medical Council (2006) *Good Medical Practice.* www.gmc-uk.org/guidance/good_medical_practice.asp

General Medical Council (2009) *Tomorrow's Doctors.*

GfK NOP Social Research (2011) *NHS Staff Tracking Research – Winter 2010* (Research Wave 5). London: Department of Health.

Glazer, BG and Strauss, AL (1967) *The Discovery of Grounded Theory: Strategies for qualitative research.* Chicago: Aldine.

Global Health Education Consortium. globalhealtheducation.org/resources/Pages/default.aspx

Godlee, F (2011) Delayed cord clamping and improved infant outcomes. *British Medical Journal*, 343: d7127.

Green, BN, Johnson, CD and Adams, A (2006) Writing narrative literature reviews for peer-reviewed journals: secrets of the trade. *Journal of Chiropractic Medicine*, 5(3): 101–17. www.ncbi.nlm.nih.gov/pmc/articles/PMC2647067

Green, B, Greene, R and Blundo, R (2009) *Gerontology and the Construction of Old Age*. New Brunswick: Aldine Transaction.

Greenhalgh, T (2010) *How to Read a Paper: The basics of evidence-based medicine*, 4th edition. London: BMJ Books/Wiley-Blackwell.

Greenhalgh, T and Peacock, R (2005) Effectiveness and efficiency of search methods in systematic reviews of complex evidence: audit of primary sources. *British Medical Journal*, 331(7524): 1064–5.

Greenhalgh, T and Russell, J (2010) Why do evaluations of ehealth programs fail? An alternative set of guiding principles. *PLoS Medicine* 7 (11): e1000360.

Greenhalgh, T, Stramer, K, Bratan, T, Byrne, E, Russell, J, Hinder, S and Potts, H (2010a) *The Devil's in the Detail: Final report of the independent evaluation of the Summary Care Record and HealthSpace programmes*. London: University College London.

Greenhalgh, T, Stramer, K, Bratan, T, Byrne, E, Russell, J and Potts, HW (2010b) Adoption and non-adoption of a shared electronic summary record in England: a mixed-method case study. *British Medical Journal*, 340: c3111.

Guba, EG and Lincoln, TS (1994) Competing paradigms in qualitative research, in Denzin, NK and Lincoln, YS (eds) *Handbook of Qualitative Research*, Beverly Hills, CA: Sage, 105–17.

Haas, PM (1992) Introduction: epistemic communities and international policy coordination. *International Organization*, 46(1): 1–35.

Haessler, S, Bhagavan, A, Kleppel, R, Hinchey, K and Visintainer, P (2012) Getting doctors to clean their hands: lead the followers. *British Medical Journal Quality and Safety* doi: 10.1136/bmjqs-2011-000396.

Hamilton, RJ and Bowers, BJ (2006) Internet recruitment and e-mail interviews in qualitative studies. *Qualitative Health Research*, 16(6): 821–35.

Hart, C (1998) *Doing a Literature Review*. London: SAGE Publications.

Haw, K and Hadfield, M (2011) *Video in Social Science Research*. London: Routledge.

Healthcare Quality Improvement Partnership (HQIP) (2009) *What is Clinical Audit?* www.hqip.org.uk/assets/Images/Uploads/HQIP-What-is-Clinical-Audit-Nov-09.pdf

Healthcare Quality Improvement Partnership (HQIP)/Cambridge Institute for Research, Education and Management (CiREM) (2011) Challenges in evaluation of quality improvement methodologies: the example of clinical audit, via link on www.hqip.org.uk/literature-on-the-effectiveness-of-clinical-audit

House of Commons Health Committee (2005) *The Prevention of Venous Thrombo-embolism in Hospitalised Patients.* HC 99. London: The Stationery Office.

Howard Hughes Medical Institute and Burroughs Wellcome Fund (2006) *Making the Right Moves: A practical guide to scientific management for postdocs and new faculty*, 2nd edition. www.hhmi.org/labmanagement.

Illich, I (1974) *Medical Nemesis.* London: Calder & Boyars.

Ilott, I, Rick, J, Patterson, M, Turgoose, C and Lacey, A (2006) What is protocol-based care? A concept analysis. *Journal of Nursing Management*, 14(7): 544–52.

Jarvis, WR (1994) Handwashing: the Semmelweis lesson forgotten? *Lancet*, 344(8933): 1311–12. www.sciencedirect.com/science/article/pii/S0140673694906874

Kass, AM and Kass, EH (1988) *Perfecting the World: The life and times of Dr. Thomas Hodgkin 1798–1866.* Boston: Harcourt Brace Jovanovich.

Kirkpatrick, DL and Kirkpatrick, JD (2006) *Evaluating Training Programs*, 3rd edition. San Francisco, CA: Berrett-Koehler.

Kohn, LT, Corrigan, JM and Donaldson, MS (eds) (2000) *To Err is Human: Building a safer health system.* Washington, DC: National Academies Press.

Krevor, BS, Ponicki, WR, Grube, JW and DeJong, W (2011) The effect of mystery shopper reports on age verification for tobacco purchases. *Journal of Health Communication*, 16(8): 820–30.

Kuhn, TS (1970) *The Structure of Scientific Revolutions*, 2nd edition. Chicago: University of Chicago Press.

Lee-Treweek, G (2000) The insight of emotional danger: research experiences in a home for older people, in Lee-Treweek, G and Linkogle, S (eds) *Danger in the Field: Risk and ethics in social research*. London: Routledge.

Leucht, S, Kissling, W and Davis, JM (2009) How to read and understand and use systematic reviews and meta-analyses. *Acta Psychiatrica Scandinavica*, 119(6): 443–50.

Lombard, M, Pastoret, PP and Moulin, AM (2007) A brief history of vaccines and vaccination. *Revue Scientifique et Technique Office International des Epizooties*, 26(1): 29–48.

McAreavey, R and Muir, J (2011) Research ethics committees: values and power in higher education. *International Journal of Social Research Methodology*, 14(5): 391–405.

McAteer, J, Stone, S, Fuller, C, Charlett, A, Cookson, B, Slade, R, Michie, S, and the NOSEC/FIT group (2008) Development of an observational measure of healthcare worker hand-hygiene behaviour: the hand-hygiene observation tool (HHOT). *Journal of Hospital Infection*, 68: 222–9.

McCulloch, J (2007) To what extent is the management of norovirus outbreaks in hospitals in the United Kingdom evidence-based? MPh dissertation, Cardiff University.

MacDermott, N, Martin, T, Nagendran, R, Nam, M, Roberts, O, Rogers, G and Rosedale, K (2005) *Coronary Heart Disease: Are the National Service Framework (NSF Wales) targets for angiography waiting times in 2004/5 being met in South Wales?* SSC report. Cardiff: Cardiff Medical School.

Macinko, JA and Starfield, B (2002) Annotated bibliography on equity in health, 1980–2001. *International Journal for Equity in Health,* 1(1): 1.

McIntyre, N and Popper, K (1983) The critical attitude in medicine: the need for a new ethics. *British Medical Journal,* 287(6409): 1919–23.

McKimm, J and Forrest, K (eds) (2011) *Professional Practice for Foundation Doctors.* Exeter: Learning Matters.

Marmot, M (2005) Social determinants of health inequalities. *Lancet* 365(9464): 1099–104.

Marsh, P and Glendenning, R (2005) *Primary Care Service Evaluation Toolkit.* www.camstrad.nhs.uk/documents/Researchers/evaluation_toolkit.pdf? preventCache=08/08/2005%2015:16 (accessed November 2010).

Maybin, J and Thorlby, R (2008) *High Quality Care for All: Briefing on NHS Next Stage Review final report. The King's Fund.* www.kingsfund.org.uk/publications/ briefings/high_quality_care.html (accessed August 2011).

Maxwell, RJ (1984) Quality assessment in health. *British Medical Journal,* 288(6428): 1470–2.

Medawar, PB (1967) *The Art of the Soluble.* London: Methuen.

Meho, LI (2006) E-mail interviewing in qualitative research: a methodological discussion. *Journal of the American Society for Information Science and Technology,* 57(10): 1284–95.

Miles, MB and Huberman, AM (1994) *Qualitative Data Analysis: An expanded sourcebook,* 2nd edition. London: Sage Publications.

Mooney, FS and Heathcote, JG (1961) Oral treatment of pernicious anaemia: further studies. *British Medical Journal,* 1(5221): 232–5.

Murdoch-Eaton, D, Drewery, S, Elton, S, Emmerson, C, Marshall, M, Smith, J, Stark, P *et al.* (2010) What do medical students understand by research and research skills? Identifying research opportunities within undergraduate projects. *Medical Teacher,* 32(3): e152–60.

Murray, CD (2004) An interpretative phenomenological analysis of the embodiment of artificial limbs. *Disability & Rehabilitation,* 26(16): 963–73.

Murray, CD and Harrison, B (2004) The meaning and experience of being a stroke survivor: an interpretative phenomenological analysis. *Disability & Rehabilitation,* 26(13): 808–16.

National Institute for Health and Clinical Excellence (NICE) (2002) *Principles for Best Practice in Clinical Audit*. Oxford: Radcliffe Medical Press.

National Institute for Health and Clinical Excellence (NICE) (2008) *Prophylaxis Against Infective Endocarditis: Antimicrobial prophylaxis against infective endocarditis in adults and children undergoing interventional procedures*. NICE clinical guideline 64. www.nice.org.uk/CG064

Nicholson, BD (2011) Research skills, in McKimm, J and Forrest, K (eds) *Professional Practice for Foundation Doctors*. Exeter: Learning Matters.

Niederstadt, C and Droste, S (2010) Reporting and presenting information retrieval processes: the need for optimizing common practice in health technology assessment. *International Journal of Technology Assessment in Health Care*, 26(4): 450–7.

Norušis, MJ (2011) *IBM SPSS Statistics 19 Guide to Data Analysis*. Upper Saddle River, NJ: Pearson.

Pickering, H, Todd, J, Dunn, D, Pepin, J and Wilkins, A (1992) Prostitutes and their clients: a Gambian survey. *Social Science & Medicine*, 34(1): 75–88.

Poland, BD (2002) Transcription quality, in Gubrium, JF and Holstein, JA (eds) *Handbook of Interview Research: Context and method*. Thousand Oaks, CA: Sage.

Popay, J, Rogers, A and Williams, G (1998) Rationale and standards for the systematic review of qualitative literature in health services research. *Qualitative Health Research*, 8(3): 341–51.

Popper, K (1959) *The Logic of Scientific Discovery*. London: Routledge.

Pugsley, L (2010) Design an effective PowerPoint presentation. *Education for Primary Care*, 21(1): 51–3.

Rabe, H, Reynolds, GJ and Diaz-Rosello, JL (2004) Early versus delayed umbilical cord clamping in preterm infants. *Cochrane Database of Systematic Reviews*, Issue 4. article no.: CD003248.

Ramsay, J, Richardson, J, Carter, YH, Davidson, LL and Feder, G (2002) Should health professionals screen women for domestic violence? Systematic review. *British Medical Journal*, 325(7359): 314.

Read, S and Maslin-Prothero, S (2011) The involvement of users and carers in health and social research: the realities of inclusion and engagement. *Qualitative Health Research*, 21(5): 704–13.

Robertson, A, Cresswell, K, Takian, A, Petrakaki, D, Crowe, S, Cornford, T, Barber, N *et al.* (2010) Implementation and adoption of nationwide electronic health records in secondary care in England: qualitative analysis of interim results from a prospective national evaluation. *British Medical Journal*, 341: c4564.

Robson, C (2000) *Small-scale Evaluation.* London: Sage Publications.

Rohde, H, Qin, J, Cui, Y, Li, D, Loman, NJ, Hentschke, M, Chen, W *et al.* (2011) Open-source genomic analysis of Shiga-toxin-producing *E. coli* O104:H4. *New England Journal of Medicine,* 365(8): 718–24.

Rossi, P, Lipsey, M and Freeman, H (2004) *Evaluation: A systematic approach.* London: Sage Publications.

Sackett, DL, Rosenberg, WMC, Gray, JAM, Haynes, RB and Richardson, WS (1996) Evidence based medicine: what it is and what it isn't. *British Medical Journal,* 312(7023): 71–2.

Sacks, H (1984) Notes on methodology, in Atkinson, JM and Heritage, J (eds) *Structures of Social Action: Studies in conversation analysis.* Cambridge: Cambridge University Press.

Schoenbach, VJ (2004) Data analysis and interpretation: concepts and techniques for managing, editing, analyzing and interpreting data from epidemiologic studies. www.epidemiolog.net/evolving/DataAnalysis-and-interpretation. pdf

Schroter, S, Black, N, Evans, S, Godlee, F, Osorio, L and Smith, R (2008) What errors do peer reviewers detect, and does training improve their ability to detect them? *Journal of the Royal Society of Medicine,* 101: 507–14.

Secretary of State for Health (2008) *High Quality Care for All.* NHS next stage review final report. CM 7432. www.dh.gov.uk/en/Healthcare/Highqualitycare-forall/index.htm

Simon, C and Mosavel, M (2010) Community members as recruiters of human subjects: ethical considerations. *American Journal of Bioethics,* 10(3): 3–11. www. ncbi.nlm.nih.gov/pmc/articles/PMC3139466/pdf/nihms212939.pdf

Sizer, AR (2007) Assessing the health and health needs of off-street male sex workers in Britain. MPH dissertation. Cardiff University.

Sobo, EJ, Bowman, C and Gifford, AL (2008) Behind the scenes in health care improvement: the complex structures and emergent strategies of implementation science. *Social Science & Medicine,* 67(10): 1530–40.

Statham, J, Mooney, A, Boddy, J and Cage, M (2011) Taking stock: a rapid review of the National Child Measurement Programme. Thomas Coram Research Unit, Institute of Education, University of London. www.dh.gov.uk/prod_consum_dh/groups/dh_digitalassets/documents/digitalasset/dh_129372.pdf

Stone, MA, Redsell, SA, Ling, JT and Hay, AD (2005) Sharing patient data: competing demands of privacy, trust and research in primary care. *British Journal of General Practice,* 55(519): 783–9.

Szreter, SRS (1984) The genesis of the Registrar General's social classification of occupations. *British Journal of Sociology,* 35(4): 523–46.

Tausig, JE and Freeman, EW (1988) The next best thing to being there: conducting the clinical research interview by telephone. *American Journal of Orthopsychiatry*, 58(3): 418–27.

ten Have, P (2007) *Doing Conversation Analysis: A practical guide,* 2nd edition. London: Sage Publications.

Tricco, AC, Tetzlaff, J and Moher, D (2011) The art and science of knowledge synthesis. *Journal of Clinical Epidemiology*, 64(1): 11–20.

Vidal-Alaball, J, Butler, CC, Cannings-John, R, Goringe, A, Hood, K, McCaddon, A, McDowell, I *et al*. (2005) Oral vitamin B12 versus intramuscular vitamin B12 for vitamin B12 deficiency. *Cochrane Database Systematic Review*, Jul 20, (3): CD004655.

Vincent, C (2010) *Patient Safety*, 2nd edition. Oxford: Wiley-Blackwell.

Waring, JJ (2009) Constructing and re-constructing narratives of patient safety. *Social Science & Medicine*, 69: 1722–31.

Watson, M, Norris, P and Granas, A (2006) A systematic review of the use of simulated patients and pharmacy practice research. *International Journal of Pharmacy Practice*, 14: 83–93.

Wilkinson, R (1996) *Unhealthy Society: The afflictions of inequality*. London: Routledge.

World Health Organization (1994) *International Statistical Classification of Diseases and Related Health Problems* (ICD-10). Geneva: WHO.

World Health Organization (2003). Quality and accreditation in health care services: a global review, in *Department of Health Service Provision*. Geneva: World Health Organization.

World Health Organization (2004) *Style Guide*. http://thailand.digitaljournals. org/community/download/6

World Health Organization (2010) Assessing and tackling patient harm: a methodological guide for data-poor hospitals. Geneva: WHO.

World Health Organization (2011) *Waist Circumference and Waist–Hip Ratio. Report of a WHO expert consultation*, Geneva, 8–11 December 2008. Geneva: WHO.

Index

Note: References in **bold** apply to the Glossary.